The Threesome Handbook

C000232315

THE Threesome HANDBOOK

A PRACTICAL GUIDE TO SLEEPING WITH THREE

Vicki Vantoch

Da Capo LIFE LONG
A Member of the Perseus Books Group

Many of the designations used by manufacturers and sellers to distinguish their products are claimed as trademarks. Where those designations appear in this book and Da Capo Press was aware of a trademark claim, the designations have been printed in initial capital letters.

Copyright © 2007 by Victoria Vantoch
Illustrations copyright © by Kaya Dzankich

All rights reserved. No part of this publication may be reproduced, stored in a retrieval system, or transmitted, in any form or by any means, electronic, mechanical, photocopying, recording, or otherwise, without the prior written permission of the publisher. Printed in the United States of America. For information, address Da Capo Press, 11 Cambridge Center, Cambridge, MA 02142.

Designed by Maria E. Torres
Set in 11 point Berkeley Book by the Perseus Books Group

Cataloging-in-Publication data for this book is available from the Library of Congress.

ISBN: 978-1-56858-333-4

Published by Da Capo Press
A Member of the Perseus Books Group
www.dacapopress.com
Note: The information in this book is true and complete to the best of our knowledge. This book is intended only as an informative guide for those wishing to know more about health issues. In no way is this book intended to replace, countermand, or conflict with the advice given to you by your own physician. The ultimate decision concerning care should be made between you and your doctor. We strongly recommend you follow his or her advice. Information in this book is general and is offered with no guarantees on the part of the authors or Da Capo Press. The authors and publisher disclaim all liability in connection with the use of this book. The names and identifying details of people associated with events described in this book have been changed. Any similarity to actual persons is coincidental.

Da Capo Press books are available at special discounts for bulk purchases in the U.S. by corporations, institutions, and other organizations. For more information, please contact the Special Markets Department at the Perseus Books Group, 2300 Chestnut Street, Suite 200, Philadelphia, PA, 19103, or call (800) 810-4145, extension 5000, or e-mail special.markets@perseusbooks.com.

10 9 8 7 6 5

Dedicated to The Honey Moon
June 2005

CONTENTS

CHAPTER 1

THREE'S COMPANY

I'm a relatively attractive chick. I wear nerdy glasses and spend a lot of time in libraries. I've had nothing surgically improved. I've never flashed a *Girls Gone Wild* video crew. I'm even married to my high school sweetheart. For most of my life, I've been somewhat of a square.

But, everyone's got a kinky side. And a few years ago, my husband and I started talking about having a threesome with another woman. The more we talked about it, the better it sounded, but when we were finally ready to try a three-way, we didn't have a clue about how to turn the fantasy into a reality.

While threesomes seem to magically materialize out of pizza deliveries in porn flicks, losing your tri-virginity isn't that simple in the real world. There aren't any church-sponsored ice cream socials for the tri-curious or mainstream relationship gurus offering seminars on three-way success. And, the jealousy and possessiveness lurking in the shadows is enough to give many three-way dreamers cold feet.

As a sex and gender historian, I've long been fascinated by historical sexual misfits who fought for their right to love and screw in unorthodox ways. But it wasn't until I wanted to try a threesome myself that I became curious about today's aspiring perverts. I couldn't find a decent threesome guidebook at the library, so I started scouring the Internet, reading biographies, and asking lots of people lots of questions. As it turns out, America is full of trisexuals eager to tell their stories.

Threesomes currently rank as America's most popular sexual fantasy, and they're becoming mainstream trendy. Three-ways have become common subplots on network TV shows, and the term *threesome* now registers more than 1.8 million hits on Google. The bottom line is most people have fantasized about threesomes but don't know how to pull them off without a hitch.

In my research I've wormed my way into diverse threesome-friendly scenes with everyone from self-identified polyamorists to trendy Hollywood partiers to decidedly untrendy Renaissance Faire buffs. I've interviewed more than a hundred threesome veterans, dabblers, and dreamers; hit swingers' clubs and erotic parties; consulted sex therapists, escorts, three-way tantra instructors, alternative relationship counselors, local sexual-freedom support groups and relationship gurus of all stripes. I've also conducted grueling personal research—testing three-way pickup lines at bars, clubs, and cuddle parties; participating in threesomes of various gender and sexuality combinations; and delving into a long-term threesome relationship so serious it involved diamonds and trips to Europe.

After plenty of bumbling, I cracked the code: I learned how to make threesomes happen, how to make them great, and even how to make them last. Based on personal experience, extensive research, expert advice, and interviews, *The Threesome Handbook* covers the A to Zs of threesomes, from wooing three-way playmates to managing jealousy to the acrobatic logistics of juggling six arms and six legs in one bed. It offers step-by-step instructions to transform even jittery tri-virgins into swaggering threesome lovers. Beyond the nuts and bolts of sex with three, this book gives the lowdown on how to create sexy and emotionally rewarding threesomes based on honesty, self-awareness, and trust.

> Our belief is that the human capacity for sex and love and intimacy is far greater than most people think—possibly infinite—and that having a lot of satisfying connections simply makes it possible for you to have a lot more.
>
> —Dossie Easton and Catherine Liszt, *The Ethical Slut*

Rock Stars Get It On Three-Way Style

At the MTV Music Awards 2003, Madonna frenched Britney Spears and Christina Aguilera on national television. The kissing trio made headlines.

Artists, Writers, and Brainiacs Swing It Three-Way Style, Too

Bloomsbury Group (1905–1944)

A group of famous artists and scholars (including writer Virginia Woolf, economist John Maynard Keynes, and author E. M. Forster) were known for "loving in triangles." These turn-of-the-century free thinkers dug open marriage, bisexuality, and three-way love affairs.

There are loads of reasons to try a threesome. You only live once, and triple hot sex is nothing to scoff at. Beyond SEX^3 and triple-snuggly cuddling, threesomes offer plenty of other perks—they're ideal for exploring bisexuality, mastering black-belt level communication skills, deepening intimacy with your primary partner, breaking passive-aggressive habits, and sampling oodles of extra love. But, most importantly . . . all the cool kids are doing it.

Three-ways come in all shapes and sizes, ranging from one-night stands with strangers to drunken "whoops" with the landlady and her electrician to passionate thirty-year threesome love affairs. Some couples opt for threesomes with clear limits (i.e., sex may be cool, but long-term intimacy may not). Others prefer to dig into more complex terrain of threesome relationships with deep emotional connections (like the trio that recently married in the Netherlands).

Whether you decide to dabble in a one-night threesome fling or a more complex trio romance, you need to know that threesomes bring up challenges, so they work best for those willing to do their homework. Threesomes call us to confront jealousy, insecurity, fear of rejection, and a host of other dark seeds inside ourselves. Three-ways can be huge growth experiences that encourage us to drop our insecurities and discover how wholly lovable we really are. And, threesomes can help pry us open and teach us to love in a new way—with less possessiveness, less ego, and less fear. Three-ways can also help couples break down their old, unhealthy relationship patterns, which can feel both freeing and scary. While bringing in a third can be dazzlingly wonderful for couples in solid relationships, it can shatter relationships that aren't strong enough to weather the bumps. So, read on, bullet-proof your relationship, then go for it.

> It was strange, soothingly strange, to be back in this big bed, this marital bed, with a third person beside us, and the three of us enveloped in frank, sensual lust. It was too good to be true.
>
> —Henry Miller

By sharing these tools with you, I hope to empower you to pursue your freaky fantasies with guts and grace. The strategies and advice laid out here offer what you need to have threesomes in whatever form suits you—from three-way flings to lasting threesome love. I've culled advice from various experts and seasoned threesome veterans, many of whom have very different approaches, and while there isn't one way that works for everyone, there are certain tools essential to making threesomes work. This book is a collection of ideas, models, techniques, and strategies for you to try. Take what works for you and discard the rest.

For those who always thought monogamy was the only route to "happily ever after," this book offers some new ways to get there. I encourage you to challenge prevailing paradigms that curtail the possibilities for sex and love. Consider this an invitation to move beyond limiting cultural stereotypes about relationships, to experiment, to play, to explore yourself, to learn where you're stuck and why, and to find out what works for you and what doesn't. And maybe, you'll uncover hotter sex and more abundant love than you ever imagined. Let tri-curious dreamers emerge from their closets and embrace their secret desires.

> We had pioneered our own relationship: its freedom, intimacy, and frankness.
>
> We had thought up the idea of the trio.
>
> —Simone de Beauvoir

WARNING! READ THIS BOOK AT YOUR OWN RISK

This book contains advice that may turn your life upside down or inside out. I take no responsibility for the effect this

Famous Threesomes in History

Anaïs Nin, Henry and June Miller

French feminist Simone de Beauvoir, philosopher Jean-Paul Sartre, and Bianca Bienenfeld

Friedrich Engels (of Marxist fame) and the Burns sisters

Surrealist painter Salvador Dali, his wife Gala, and various young men

Film star Marlene Dietrich, her husband Rudi, and novelist Erich Maria Remarque

Beat poets Neil Cassady and Jack Kerouac, plus Neil's wife Carolyn

Sex researcher Alfred Kinsey, Mrs. Kinsey, and their lab assistant

Pablo Picasso, surrealist poet Paul Éluard, and his wife Maria Benz

First Lady Eleanor Roosevelt and her lesbian lovers Nancy Cook and Marion Dickerman

book has on your current or future relationships. If you aspire to radically reinvent your ho-hum life and traverse new sex and love terrain, this book is for you. In taking the steps described here, you will find yourself in unknown territory and it may scare the hell out of you. In the process of deconstructing your social programming, you may be forced to change the way you think about yourself and love in general. Indeed, in your quest for the holy grail of sex, you may discover that you've been endowed with miraculous new powers. If you're willing to take the red pill, read on.

CHAPTER 2

DARE TO DREAM: FANTASIZING YOUR WAY TO A THREESOME

Tasha and I had spent many a night detailing our desire for a threesome, even going into elaborate detail about what we'd like to do with our mystery woman who would join us in our bed. But . . . we'd never quite found the perfect person to join us. But it seemed our luck had changed, and I summoned Tasha over to me and whispered in her ear, "Baby, what do you think about Anna joining us in bed?" "You must have read my mind—as I was putting the lotion on her, I was getting so turned on. Let me feel her out and see if she's up for it," she whispered

> back. . . . Then, before I knew it, she had climbed on top of Anna. The two were laughing and then making out, their mouths pressed together as I watched. After a few minutes, they both got up, holding hands as they approached me. . . . No words were spoken as Tasha began licking my cock. . . . [Then] Anna straddled my wife's face and lowered her pussy to her mouth. . . . It was the perfect arrangement for everyone, and I kept my gaze locked on Anna as we shared the woman I love in the most intimate way.
>
> —Mr. Zachary D., British Columbia,
> letter to *Penthouse,* December 2006

Whether inspired by *Penthouse* magazine or watching Madonna, Britney, and Christina french kiss on YouTube, chances are you've probably indulged in a three-way fantasy. There's a good reason for this: threesomes are smokin' hot. And, if you want to have a real-life threesome, fantasies are the perfect place to start. So, before you start prowling craigslist for willing thirds, dig into your imagination, explore your three-way fantasies, talk three-way smut to your lover, and test your partner's tri-curiosity.

> Threesomes ranked as America's number-one sexual fantasy in a recent ABC poll.

VOCABULARY BUILDER

Tri-curious

Hot for three-way fantasies and eager to try a real-life threesome

WHAT GETS YOU WET?

Start testing your tri-curiosity with your largest sex organ: your brain. Assemble a basic threesome fantasy kit (porn magazines, saucy flicks, and erotic stories). Then, spend a Saturday afternoon spanking the monkey with a threesome scenario in mind. Who are the main characters? Two guys? Two gals? A friend? A stranger? The UPS guy? A tucked and plucked porn star? Which three-way scenario sends you rocketing to bliss? Are you itching to watch or to be watched? Are you pining to be the center of attention or a coconspirator pouncing on a third? Are you hankering to try same-sex lovin'?

My biggest fantasy is having sex with two guys. They would bathe me, shave my pussy, massage me, feed me . . . then fuck me. They wouldn't have to do anything to each other. It would all be about me. My boyfriend has finally agreed, but I haven't found the right guy.

—Brooke, 34

I had fantasized about watching my wife fuck another guy for years. When I finally watched her lick another guy's cock, I got rock hard! I found it hotter than I had even imagined.

—Eric, 38

Ten Telltale Signs That You Aspire to Have a Threesome

1. Sexy couples make you hard.
2. When your ex kisses his main squeeze, you get turned on instead of jealous.
3. When you're making out with someone, you talk dirty about an imaginary third.
4. You've jerked off while imagining two beautiful women servicing you.
5. You search personal ads for horny couples.
6. When your boyfriend brings up having a three-way, you get wet.
7. Your favorite movie is *Henry and June*.
8. You always bring a friend with you on dates.
9. You wish your boyfriend could be in two places at once.
10. When you're drunk, you make out with your two best friends.

TESTING THE WATERS: DIRTY TALK 101

Once you know what wets your knickers, mention it to your beau in a steamy moment. If he gets his rocks off, you've planted a Pavlovian seed. If he doesn't take to it, you'll have to lay a little more groundwork. Start by talking dirty. Watch for your lover's reaction. If he's into it, keep going. If you're new to dirty talk, use terms that don't make you bust out laughing. (There's no need to jump into "hot throbbing cock" talk if that isn't your thing). Keep it simple: tell your lover what you want the third person to do, who the third person would be, and other details about the scenario. If your lover isn't into it, try an instant revision. Maybe your lover got sidetracked wondering if the third party was a better lover. Sometimes a new cast or a new setting is enough to hit a lover's magic three-way button. If your lover still isn't biting, try asking him to tell you about his threesome fantasy.

I slept with this guy, who asked me to tell him about my threesome fantasies. I told him about how I wanted to be with him and another guy from our class. While we were having sex, he asked me to describe the fantasy in detail. I told him how the two of them would lick me all over and penetrate me at the same time. He was so turned on by the whole thing and so was I. That was the best sex I've ever had. And, I've wanted to try a threesome ever since.

—Bekki, 24

Pavlov's Three-Way Training

Remember Pavlov and his dogs? If your lover doesn't immediately get hard over your threesome fantasy, use Pavlov's training technique to cultivate your lover's three-way urge. Talk dirty about a threesome while performing world-class tongue technique. Pamper him. Love him just the way he likes it. Keep talking about a threesome. Repeat as necessary. With any luck, he'll develop an association between sexual nirvana and threesomes.

I didn't have any three-way fantasies until my boyfriend started talking dirty to me about bringing in another woman. At first, it didn't do much for me. Then I noticed that every time I played with myself, I fantasized about having a threesome. That's when I realized I wanted to try it, but I wasn't sure how far I'd be willing to go or how far I was willing to let him go with another woman. So, I stuck to fantasies and talking dirty about it, until I felt confident about it. By the time we actually tried it, we had been talking about it and fantasizing about it for ages, so it was a major turn-on.

—Kim, 33

If your lover seems upset at the mere mention of a threesome, talk about it. Pressure tactics tend to lead to disappointing threesome experiences. So, instead of whining to get your way, try being patient, honest, and communicative. If you're in a committed, long-term relationship and you can honestly offer reassurance, do it. Tell him he fulfills you. Ask him how he feels about exploring threesome fantasies together without any expectation or pressure that it'll actually happen. If he okays this, keep playing with threesome dirty talk until he feels comfortable enough to start considering the possibility of trying a real threesome. If he still refuses, dump him and steal his cash.

Threesome Flicks

Summer Lovers (1982)
Peter Gallagher and Daryl Hannah star in a film about an emotional and sexual triad relationship in Greece.

Threesome (1994)
A love triangle of three college roommates (two guys and a woman).

Three of Hearts (1993)
A romantic comedy starring Kelly Lynch and William Baldwin, about a love triangle between a straight cad, his lesbian best friend, and her former lover (a bisexual woman).

Wild Things 2 (2004)
An insurance investigator becomes involved with two young women.

American Psycho (2000)
The film's lead has a threesome with two female escorts.

Wild Things (1998)
Denise Richards, Neve Campbell, and Matt Dillon engage in a steamy threesome.

Kinsey (2004)
American sexologist Alfred Kinsey, his wife, and their lab assistant become sexually involved.

Two Girls and a Guy (1997)
Two women find they're dating the same guy (Robert Downey, Jr.).

Jules et Jim (1962)
Two friends (Jules and Jim) fall in love with the same woman; they find love and friendship.

Sunday Bloody Sunday (1971)
A threesome between a gay man, a straight woman, and a bi man.

Café au Lait (1993)
A French woman living in Paris gets pregnant by one of her two lovers, and the three form a family.

Farinelli (1994)
A young castrati has a ménage à trios with his less-talented composer brother.

Design for Living (1933)
Two Americans sharing an apartment in Paris fall for the same woman.

French Twist (1995)
A philandering real estate agent and his wife are changed when the wife invites a lesbian to live with them.

Heart Beat (1980)
Beat poets Jack Kerouac and Neal Cassady have a threesome with Neal's wife Carolyn.

Henry and June (1990)
Writer Henry Miller and his wife June become romantically involved with Anaïs Nin.

Paint Your Wagon (1969)
Lee Marvin and Clint Eastwood play partners living in Gold Rush–era California, where they start a town and share a wife.

Underworld: Evolution (2006)
A hot vampire threesome (two female vamps and a man) takes place, as the vampires and werewolves battle for domination.

Quinceañera (2006)
A Mexican-American man has an all-male threesome with his neighbors, a long-term couple.

Three of Hearts: A Postmodern Family (2004)
A documentary of a triad relationship between two guys and a woman.

Shortbus (2006)
A group of New Yorkers gather at an underground salon for bawdy sex and art; featuring an all-male threesome.

Hot Threesome Tales to Get You Started

I was teaching an art class and my TA told me that she always wanted to be with a woman. For over twenty years, she'd been thinking about it. As a little graduation present after the class, I told her I had a surprise for her. I had called the woman I was dating, (who was bi) and told her to get naked, lay on her bed at a certain time, and blindfold herself. She agreed to do it. . . . I drove her to my girlfriend's place and on the way, I said I had arranged a nice fantasy. When we got there, I took the TA by the hand and led her into my girlfriend's place. I told her that I wanted her to have the opportunity to live out her fantasy and I took her into the bedroom, where my girlfriend was lying naked on the bed. She went over and sat down. I introduced them. She was nervous, but also thrilled. I could tell. Soon, the TA was caressing my girlfriend's legs, hips, stomach, breasts, and my girlfriend was enjoying it. Then, my TA did something I didn't expect. She asked me if I could leave the room. I smiled and said, "of course." And, I did. I did watch through the crack in the door, however, and it was quite exciting to watch someone live out a twenty-year fantasy. Still I would have loved to stay in the room. Damn.

—Mike, 35

I usually only date bi women because I love threeways so much. It's amazing to have a chance to live out a fantasy that you've seen in pornos hundreds of times. I dated this one woman who used to invite her friends over for us to fuck (yeah, she pretty much kicked ass). One night we were having a three-way with one of her friends. I was fucking her friend from behind, while she was eating out my girlfriend. I pulled out to cum and my girlfriend sat up, put my cock in her mouth and I came in it. That was probably the single most amazing thing that's ever happened to me, sexually or otherwise, and I *still* love her for that.

—Darius, 24

My boyfriend and I met this sexy, smart woman at a friend's party. She flirted with me. I asked her if she liked girls. She just gave a naughty smile. I was dying to touch her. My boyfriend came over and started joking with her. I told her I wanted to see them kiss. They started kissing and it was so damned hot. We brought her home and stayed up all night.

—Ashley, 31

Saturday Night: A True Story

by Hannah H.

As a chick, I always got turned on watching threesome porn scenes with D, but I wasn't sure I'd enjoy it in real life. Until . . . It all started innocently enough at a dinner party at a friend's house. Sexy stories and many drinks later, D and I were on the couch, kissing and getting naked. His cock was out and hard. Moving down, I rested my head on his stomach and took him in hand and mouth. I loved the sensation of rubbing my wet lips over the silkiness of his head, softly, slowly, back and forth. Other people wandered around the room, but I was oblivious, totally getting into D and his cock.

Our friend H sat down beside us, slowly stroking himself. Relaxed and excited, ready for something different, I looked at H's cock. Both men waited to see what I would do, neither speaking or moving. Would two hard cocks be too much for me? There was only one way to find out. As I moved down, I kept a hand on D, discovering H's skin and scent with my mouth. Looking up at one then the other, I kept rubbing, licking, and sucking them. And they stared back, their eyes low and shaded with pleasure and excitement. At that moment, kneeling between them, did I feel manipulated or threatened? No. With a cock in each hand, I was in control of them. Their pleasure was mine to give, take, and direct.

I moved back and forth between them, filling my mouth with D's cock while stroking H. Then switching. And again. I was no longer thinking about either man. They were simply cocks for me to play with and use as I pleased. Turning my head back and forth, back and forth, I suddenly needed them to be closer together. "Lie next to each other." Obediently, they shifted—shoulder to shoulder, hip to hip. I grabbed both their cocks, pulling them together so they touched each other. I lowered my mouth, filling myself with two hard cocks, feeling each slide against the other over my tongue, under my tongue, inside my hot mouth. I was wet. I felt kinky. I was out of my head, just going for it. It was awesome.

D and H loved it, of course. How could they not? Whether either gave a thought to how they were touching each other—cock to cock, balls squeezed together—seemed irrelevant with me on top. And since it turned me on, I knew they had to be turned on, too. We shifted then again. D moved to fuck me from behind, while I took H's cock in my mouth. And just like the pornos, the men switched places. Intense, mindless fucking, so pleasurable that I felt like one huge wet, open pussy.

An Erotic Three-Way Tale: Midnight Seduction

by R. Pia

"I want to taste you," Alexis commanded, her guttural tone rasping with desire as she gazed over Kaarina's supple curves. Kaarina obediently straddled Alexis's face. Slick, wet lips met hers and she parted them to find the bundled nerves of the girl's clitoris. Engulfed in the sensual scent of female, she hummed against Kaarina's clean-shaven vulva and stuck two fingers into her core, eliciting a wanton wiggle of her hips. Silky thighs brushed her ears with each stroke of her tongue. Justin watched mesmerized.

Kneeling, Justin pulled the curve of Kaarina's hips towards his pelvis. Alexis watched from below, as he brushed and teased his shaft against Kaarina's bottom. Alexis gave one bated breath into Kaarina's core as Justin slipped inside her. Alexis felt the meticulous rhythm of each thrust as she continued licking Kaarina's petals, moist with desire. The young man's slick shaft glistened in the candlelight as he slid in and out of Kaarina's creamy walls. Kaarina's whimpers grew toward impending bliss, rousing Alexis's senses. Justin's tempo increased until he withdrew to ejaculate, his milky essence completely covered the henna tattoo at the base of Kaarina's spine. Alexis then circled the mushroom head of his cock and licked away the remaining drops of his pearly seed. The taste of male and female lined her lips and she lapped at it hungrily.

GEARING UP

Just because three-way visions bring you to the edge every time, that doesn't mean the reality will pan out the same way. You could be pleasantly surprised or disappointed.

The taste of pussy might disgust you in fantasyland and leave you dripping wet in reality (or vice versa). And, sometimes, threesome fantasies might be all you need—for one, imaginary third parties are exceptionally obedient and rarely inspire jealous pangs. And not all relationships can handle introducing a third and not all individuals are secure enough to share a lover. So, if you're in a committed relationship and your lover isn't ready for a real threesome, stick to fantasyland until you're both totally onboard. Give your lover plenty of time to warm up to the idea. (Dirty talk isn't too shabby, is it?) Your lover may never want to try a threesome, but, many people are eager to try a three-way under the right conditions. So, it's your job to set up the right conditions. Proceed to the next chapter to find out how. . . .

VOCABULARY BUILDERS

Cheating

So 1997, so uncool.

Closed relationship

Old-fashioned monogamy.

Daytona Beach three-way

A three-way featuring two drunk women, dyking out to impress the boys.

Don't ask, don't tell

A committed relationship in which partners can screw around discreetly.

Ethical slut

A nonmonogamist, who becomes emotionally and/or sexually involved with more than one person with honesty and mutual consent. The term comes from *The Ethical Slut,* by Dossie Easton and Catherine Lizt, the fairy godmothers of hipster nonmonogamy.

Open relationship

A relationship in which both agree to extracurricular sexual activity, either together or individually.

Polyamory

Coined in the late 1990s, the term literally means "many loves." Poly people have more than one romantic relationship simultaneously (with honesty). Contrary to swingers, polyamorists aren't just in it to schtoop strangers: they're in it for love (aw).

Tri-phobia

A fear of or moral opposition to threesome sex and relationships. They're likely to exclaim, "That's sick!" (May be the result of repressed trisexual urges.)

Party trisexual

Someone who only participates in threesome sex after several martinis.

Triad

A threesome relationship that involves sex and emotional connection.

Trinogamous

A committed threesome relationship, with no extracurricular nooky.

Trisexual

The sexual orientation of a person who prefers sex with two partners simultaneously.

Lifestyle trisexual

Couples and singles who only indulge in threesome flings with no emotional strings attached.

Vee

A threesome, in which one person has sex with two lovers, who aren't into each other sexually. . . . Think one straight girl with two straight guys, *capice*?

Three-Way Fantasy Exercises

1. Flip through your favorite porn magazine; cut out threesome images that make you hot.
2. Flirt with a couple. Go home. Picture them kissing you. Stick your hand down your pants.
3. Watch a threesome-centric porn flick with your lover, tickle her pearl during the steamy scenes.
4. Read your lover a story from *Three-way: Erotic Stories* by Alison Tyler.
5. Tell your lover a threesome fantasy, while performing first-rate oral sex on him.

CHAPTER 3

THE MATING^3 GAME: FINDING THE PERFECT TRI-LOVERS

I met this very attractive man at an office party. We had a few drinks together. He asked me if I had a boyfriend, I said no. I asked if he had a girlfriend. He said yes. I thought, *Shit.* Then, he mentioned that they had an open relationship. Next, he asked me if I liked women. I wouldn't give him that satisfaction, so I just didn't answer. Then his girlfriend showed up at the party and she looked like a Victoria's Secret model. She was fucking gorgeous. I immediately texted him from across the room: "Yes, I definitely like girls!" He texted back: "Do you want to come to

> our place?" I texted back: "Yes, but I'm not sure she's into me." He texted: "I'll check." Then, they both walked over and kidnapped me for the night. It was fantastic. The next day, I felt like a fucking rock star.
>
> —Yva, 27

Okay, you've spent enough time in fantasyland and you're ready to hit the streets, now what? Threesomes can be initiated just about anywhere—from bars to bible groups. When it comes down to it, nearly everyone is tri-curious, so consider the world your oyster. But, prepare to kick it up a notch because starting a threesome requires extra attitude, extra confidence, and extra style. You'll need to find the hotspots for meeting three-way lovers, choose the right threesome playmates, and seduce your ideal third. This chapter is divided into three sections, dedicated to the who, where, and how of three-way pickup.

Warning: If your partner is still fuming at the mention of a three-way, *do not* attempt to pick up a third. No matter how randy you're feeling, a three-way ambush isn't an effective strategy. Return to Dirty Talk 101 (page 13) and review communication strategies (chapter 4).

WHO'S YOUR DREAM THREE-WAY LOVER?

There's nothing less sexy than having a three-way with someone who flips out the next day or starts crying during a three-way daisy chain. Sure, it's possible to squash someone's internal conflict through a series of savvy seduction strategies and a bottle of tequila, but it's not worth it if your hookup can't live with the consequences. Threesomes require more sexual openness and emotional maturity than sex with two, and getting involved with partners who can't handle it can be a direct route to tears and tantrums. A kinky night isn't worth a boiled bunny on the doorstep. Plus, sex is way hotter when everyone involved feels great about what they're doing.

So, don't settle for the wrong three-way playmates just because they're willing and you're scared you'll never have the chance again. Three-way desperation is lame. Have an abundance mentality. Plenty of people are tri-curious and open to sexual exploration, so there's no need to seduce someone who's likely to regret it, blame you, or try to break up your relationship. Know the truth about threesomes: most people have fantasized about having one and many are itchin' to try it. So, put in the effort to find the right partners.

While threesome veterans all look for different qualities in three-way lovers, their success hinges on having clear personal standards about who they're willing to schtoop in a three-way and a willingness to walk away if the situation or playmates don't meet their standards. Threesome enthusiasts say that three-ways work best when there's minimal rivalry, competitiveness, possessiveness, and jealousy. When asked what qualities they seek in threesome lovers, interviewees' lists included: balanced giver/taker, openly bisexual, confident, free of sexual hang-ups, good communicator, comfortable with living an unconventional life, thoughtful lover, and nonpossessive.

Couples need to pay special attention to three-way playmate selection because certain thirds can jeopardize relationships. What constitutes a "safer" playmate varies for every couple, depending on their goals and fears. By discussing threesome-related insecurities in advance, couples can negotiate how to choose safer three-way playmates. Many couples nix anyone either member feels might threaten their relationship. Some couples prefer to hire sex workers (because there's no threat of a burgeoning romance), some only invite trusted friends, and others feel safest seducing a third at a sex party (because there's less chance of emotional attachment). Smokin' good looks may be all that matters for couples scoring one night three-way flings at sex parties, where there's no expectation of future contact.

True Tales

Seasoned trio lovers give the scoop on choosing playmates

My boyfriend and I had a threesome with a friend. She flirted with us, kissed us, and we ended up having wild sex. She loved fucking my boyfriend; she was totally into it; she came a zillion times while I was licking her pussy. Then she totally freaked out. She said she wasn't really gay and she shouldn't be fucking my boyfriend. She was really confused. That was her trip. She's got religious parents and she's got a lot of guilt. My boyfriend and I vowed never to have sex with her again. When people start experimenting, sometimes they freak out about what they find. It's not worth it to have sex with someone who's going to feel bad about it later or realize she's Christian or get scared that she likes pussy so much. Now, I only have three-ways with women when I know they can handle it. They're way more fun now that we choose the right women.

—Lori, 29

My partner and I don't get involved with overly jealous or possessive people because we've dealt with the drama that comes along with that.

—Yvonne, 27

I feel good about bringing another woman in if I get the vibe that I can trust her—I just need to feel confident that she's not interested in getting into a relationship with my guy.

—Anna, 25

I'm picky about who I invite into the bedroom with my boyfriend. I only have threesomes with women who are easygoing, bisexual (and comfortable with it), noncompetitive, communicative, and low drama. Friends with too much baggage (no matter how attractive and eager to try a threesome) are out of bounds.

—Beth, 35

Previous threesome experience required . . .
I don't get romantically involved with anyone who doesn't have experience with ethical non-monogamy, because I don't want to spend the time and energy to teach the skills necessary and to work through all the social programming to help them come to terms with an alternative lifestyle. It's too much work.

—Christos, who has lived in a triad for eight years

Drawing the line at insanity . . .
I just don't get into threesomes with anyone so crazy that they interfere with my life or the lives of those around me.

—Kay, 37

Yogi Three-Way Says: Know the Universal Law of Attraction

Ask and ye shall receive. Trust that the universe will offer whatever you request, once you put your own house in order. Once you've developed a list of qualities you seek in three-way lovers, notice if your list contains qualities that you yourself possess. Maybe your list of the perfect lover contains qualities you'd like to develop in yourself. Develop these qualities in yourself first. If you seek a good communicator, become a good communicator. The universal law of attraction will magnetize good communicators to you. It might sound too hippie-dippy for you, but relationship gurus report that like attracts like. Set your intention to meet someone who at least matches your own vibration.

Threesome Decoder Key

(B)F^2M = 2 bi females + 1 straight male

(G)MMF = 1 gay male + 1 straight male + 1 straight female

(B)M^2F = 2 bi males + 1 straight female

(B)FFM = 1 bi female + 1 straight female + 1 straight male

(G)F^3 = 3 gay females

(G)M^3 = 3 gay males

F^2M = 2 straight females + 1 straight male

M^2F = 2 straight males + 1 straight female

CONSIDER THE OPTIONS

Gay, bisexual, bi-curious, bi-comfortable, or straight playmates

How gay will you play? If you're in it for the gay exploration, consider the options: (B)F^2M, (B)FFM, (G)FFM, (G)MMF, (B)M^2F, M^2F, (B)F^3, (G)F^3, (G)F^2F, (G)F. There's nothing more wondrous than having a hang-up-free, gay, or bi lover usher you into the joys of gay sex. Plus, for squeamish and fearful first-timers, having a gay guide means you can lay back and let them please you first, until you're ready to try it yourself. Also, many green gay adventurers find that it's much less fun to swing it with uncomfortable bi-curious lovers, who've got their own homophobia and shame to contend with. Many openly bisexual women say sleeping with straight women requires extra energy to manage sexual orientation meltdowns (which usually surface after or during a night of exquisite gay sex in a trio). Even in the era of gay pride, first gay encounters often evoke shame, fear, and guilt. Kudos to the veteran bisexuals and homosexuals, who enjoy initiating straighties. One thirty-one-year-old bisexual woman said:

> I'm openly bisexual and I only choose confident, comfortable bisexual women for threesomes. I used to sleep with straight women who were experimenting, but I found that being the initiator takes

> too much energy, and it's a recipe for chaos. I don't want to have to walk straight women through the whole process of sexual identity confusion. I find that it's just easier to have sex with women who have already gone through that process and feel comfortable with their sexuality.

But, gay guides aren't ideal for all novice gay-sex dabblers. Some first timers feel best experimenting with straight people of the same sex because it feels . . . well, straighter. Straight American men seem to get their panties in a knot about guy-on-guy action, so many guys prefer threesomes with other self-identified straight guys because it defuses the scary prospect of gay sexual contact. Threesomes with two straight guys can be a good gateway to same-sex exploration for men because it allows them to get comfortable being naked and turned-on in the vicinity of another guy. Once the comfort level develops, some straight American guys find themselves more willing to go further with same-sex action and up for experimenting with gay or openly bisexual men.

For those who fantasize more about watching and being watched than bi-curious experimentation, straight three-way playmates may be ideal. A threesome with two straight members might resemble a vee, rather than a balanced threesome. (A vee is when one person gets it on with two people, who aren't that attracted to each other.)

Straight people hankering for exhibitionist or voyeuristic delights often find vees sublime.

Raw three-way sex versus threesomes with heart

Some couples seek three-ways for pure sexual fun, while others seek emotional intimacy with thirds. In this model, the couple seeks three-way flings. The goal: sticking it to someone new without any emotional involvement. Couples interested in sexual variety or getting their bisexual freak on may find sex-only three-ways ideal. Sure, insecurities may bubble up, but many people find that this type of threesome is the easiest to manage and doesn't require as much of a start-up investment in communication as other threesome models. The goal is sex play, plain, and simple. And, the role of the third is clear cut: sex toy.

Couples seeking sex-only threesomes are very clear about not wanting to get involved in a complex relationship with another person, so they're careful not to intertwine their social lives with three-way sexual expeditions. These couples create strict limits about their playmates to keep the three-way adventures solely sexual (for some, friends are strictly off-limits.) That way, if things get sticky, they can quickly extricate the third party without maintaining any social ties or long-term contact. These couples generally pick their thirds from the enormous pool of hotties at sex parties, online meet-ups, and other erotic venues. Sex-oriented threesomes can last anywhere from a night to months.

Other couples, however, dig more complex, emotional connections with the third party. They're up for the additional intimacy and companionship of another lover. These trio lovers prefer to develop intense trio relationships and they're more likely to get romantically involved with friends and people they meet through polyamory networks. One twenty-eight-year-old male grad student who's been romantically involved with a straight couple for nine months, said:

> I get to know people for at least a few months before becoming sexually involved. It's a requirement for me to know the person. I have no interest in being a couple's boy toy. A lot of people want to be used for sex, but I'm not like that. I've done that, and it just doesn't interest me anymore. I need the emotional satisfaction. The relationships are important to me.

The weirdness factor: Deciding whether to fondle friends or strangers

Knowing whether you're after no-strings-attached three-way booty or a potentially more complex emotional connection might inform whether you're up for sleeping with friends. Obviously, threesomes with friends can put the friendship at risk. Couples getting involved with friends need to consider whether they're both willing to sever the friendship if things get hairy. Some couples into sex-only threesomes never fuck friends: "My wife and I never have threesomes with friends. That's our rule. I like to keep my friends. It could be a rotten experience, and then we'd have to deal with awkwardness. I don't want that. Awkwardness isn't fun. I don't want my threesomes to turn into anything other than fun. So, as soon as it's not fun, it's over."

But, sometimes three-way friend shagging is worth the risk. Threesomes with close friends can be damned magical, especially when everyone's on the same page in terms of expectations and boundaries. One woman who's had threesomes with friends put it this way: "Threesomes with friends can cause problems, but the connection, trust, and experience can be much better if you do embark with a friend. Plus, would you pass on a thrilling toboggan ride because you might hit a pothole?" Wendy-O Matic, author of *Redefining Our Relationships*, who has been living in alternative relationships for years, says her romances always begin with friendship:

> An equally disheartening misconception is the old adage "Intimacy or sex will ruin the friendship." This is certainly true if you haven't established a

> good foundation of trust and communication with this friend or if you never really had a commitment to the friendship in the first place. Every lover has always been my friend first. If you set out to communicate and understand your expectations (reasonable and otherwise) with your friends, then you may be surprised by the potential of a friendship to evolve into something more intimate or more sexual or more emotionally bonding. Keep in mind that sex is only one of the million ways to express love. . . . The new adage should be "Intimacy with a friend means never having to break up, because you know that you're still friends the next day."

Another bonus of choosing friends for your trio is that you probably already know their shit. You probably know which friends are inclined to instigate extra drama in their lives—(you've seen them berate boyfriends, break bottles in jealous fits, or leave drunk messages at three AM). You probably have a good idea of how they handle their romantic relationships and how they feel about sex. And, knowing someone's dark side can be a good thing. If your friend meets your personal standards for three-way playmates and you're all in agreement about expectations and boundaries, a friend-based threesome might be just what the doctor ordered.

WARNING SIGNS: IDENTIFYING AND BOOTING DESTRUCTIVE THIRDS

Some couples protect their relationship from destructive thirds by agreeing to a come-between rule in advance. This rule grants each member of the couple veto power over a threesome playmate if either member of the couple feels the third is threatening their relationship. Stephane Hemon, a seduction guru who's had several one to three month threesomes with his girlfriend of three years said, "We have a rule that if anyone ever tries to come between us, that person is out. Couples have to set up that rule right from the beginning. You can usually feel it in your solar plexus, you can feel it when someone has a hidden agenda." Knowing that your partner will cut off contact with the third party if you make the request can help both members of the couple feel much safer about three-way fun. A lawyer who's been married for eighteen years and has had numerous threesomes with his bisexual wife described their veto rule:

> Single bi chicks playing with couples tend to be a little needy; they tend to want threesomes to be about them. That's fine. That's partly what's attractive about it, to focus on one person. But, when the person tries to come between us, and that happens all the time, we just end it. If my wife says heave ho, I agree. It's fairly simple, because we never play with

friends so we're not tied into doing other social activities with the person.

It's not always easy to identify potentially destructive and pain-in-the-ass three-way lovers, so watch for these red flags:

Warning: Beware of Conflicted Three-Way Lovers

Choose willing and eager three-way partners. Follow one simple rule: don't pressure anyone into it. Steer clear of anyone reluctant or conflicted about having a threesome. Threesomes misfire most when someone is cajoled into it before they're ready. Take license to flirt your booty off, run chemistry checks with potential three-way playmates, tell your target that you're up for a three-way, or rub baby oil all over yourself—just don't be so desperate for a threesome that you resort to lame manipulation tactics. If someone seems conflicted about it, they'll likely get "buyer's remorse" and pull you into an emotional tailspin. Be willing to walk away.

Warning: Beware of Triangulators

Triangulators can swiftly transform a happy trio dynamic into a deadly love triangle, the threesome's ugly cousin. Triangulators incite rivalry or jealousy to get what they want. They're often insecure people who use three-ways to bolster their emaciated self-worth. Nip triangulation in the bud—either call the triangulator out on it and work through the issue, or send the triangulator packing.

Warning Signs: Talking or complaining to one person about problems with the third, instead of approaching the person directly; asking one person to keep secrets from another; pressuring one member of the couple to develop more intimacy (without discussing it with the other member of the couple).

Warning: Beware of Attention Whores

Focusing attention on someone new can be part of what makes a threesome hot, but the best three-way lovers don't hog all the affection. Sure, an established couple will need to make the new person feel extra welcome, but picking a third who's balanced in terms of giving and receiving makes it much more fun for everyone. And, those who need too much attention may end up being too draining. Watch for thirds who take love from both members of the couple and give little back.

Warning Signs: The third delivers an unprompted five-hour monologue and expects you both to listen attentively; this type may also expect you to pick up the tab for everything and to pony up 14-karat gifts.

Others to Avoid in Three-Ways

Devout Catholics: Brimming with built-in homophobia and sex shame, these guiltmongers have a strong hunch that nonprocreative sex is morally suspect.

Squares: They're obsessed with white picket fences and deeply dazzled by monogamy; plus, they're still trying to please their parents and the Joneses.

Homophobes: They're still wondering whether homosexuality is a medical affliction.

Drama Queens: Insisting on center stage, they thrive on the adrenaline rush from emotional turmoil and relish stoking conflict. They may also seek constant reassurance and affection in the form of flattery and gifts.

Competitors: They delight in competition and rivalry.

Loners: They lack friends and have never had a long-term, healthy relationship.

Trio Playmate Profiles

The experimentalist/artist/free spirit/seeker/rebel and rocker

Free thinkers, who prefer independence to social conformity and eschew labels altogether

Pros: They won't flinch at alternative sexual experiences or long-term romances.

Cons: N/A

How to spot them: Piercing, tatts, bright pink hair, and fluorescent poodles

Where to spot them: Hip art shows, costume parties, and WTO protests

The self-identified bisexual

The holy grail of threesome sex

Pros: They dig chicks and dudes.

Cons: Competition—they're in high demand.

How to spot them: They'll tell you in a flash.

Where to spot them: They're everywhere.

The seasoned polyamorist

Self-identified polyamorists who date multiple lovers simultaneously with honesty and consent

Pros: An honest, no-nonsense approach to communication

Cons: The overly earnest communication style may fizzle the magic of seduction.

How to spot them: Sarcasm-free conversations

Where to spot them: Ren Faire and Sci-Fi conventions

The newly single

Divorcees and jilted lovers seeking an ego boost after a wilted marriage or soured love affair

Pros: They're up for three-ways with couples for the double dose of affection.

Cons: They require too much attention.

How to spot them: Low-cut shirts, a bottle of booze, a posse of friends, and divorce papers.

Where to spot them: Straight bars and other square venues.

The tantric lover

Old-school tantra vixens, renowned for their radical lovestyles

Pros: They're open to "merging with more than one soul" and skilled at multiple orgasms, ejaculation control, and other sexual perks.

Cons: Pillow talk likely to run seven to ten hours with a heavy focus on chakras, healing, "triadic consciousness," and yonis (that's hippie for "crotch"). Not recommended for busy professionals.

How to spot Them: Nicknames like Twin Flame and Iguana's Breath.

Where to spot them: Clothing-optional resorts, tantric sex workshops, pagan ceremonies, raw-food eateries, and ashrams.

The fireball

Charismatic, magnetic types who draw people in

Pros: The roller-coaster ride. These attention-magnets are apt to jump in the sack with couples for the rush.

Cons: The roller-coaster ride. They're likely to turn your life inside out once you sleep with them. (Have a therapist on call to rescue you from the crazy-maker vortex.)

How to spot them: They're the center of attention at any party.

Where to spot them: Wherever they're most likely to be seen

LOOKING TO THE STARS: ASTROLOGY FOR THREE-WAY MATCHES

Still stumped about how to choose the right three-way lovers? Review the charts for hot threesome combinations. Those who share the same astrological element make compatible friends and lovers. Opposite elements on the zodiac wheel also spark magic.[1]

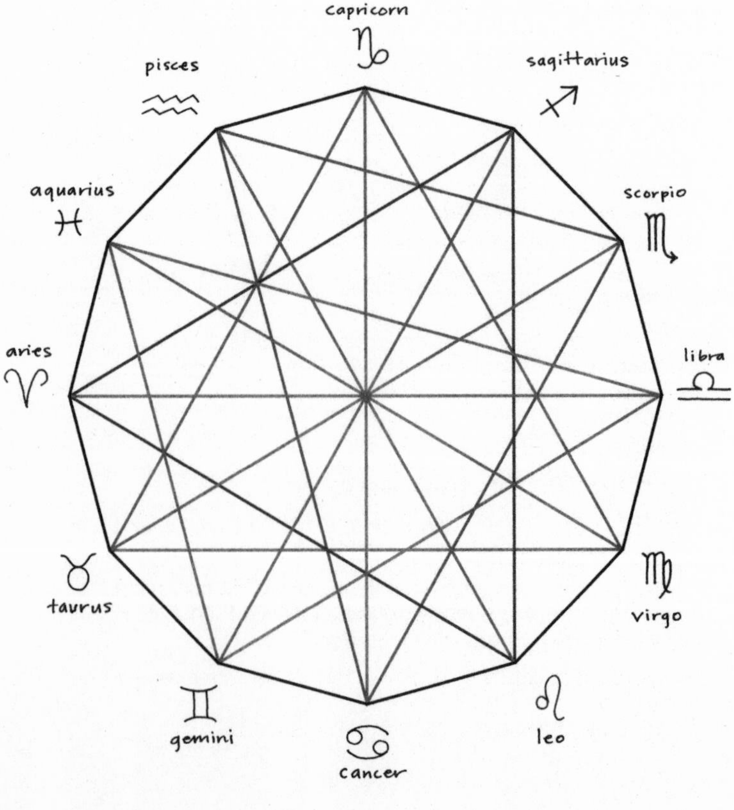

Aquarius (January 20–February 19)
A lack of jealousy and an inquisitive, freedom-loving nature makes an ideal candidate for threesomes and bisexuality. Aquarius has a deep desire to overturn the status quo and welcomes the challenges of unconventional lifestyles. Three-ways are likely to win Aquarius over if there's ample mental stimulation and her freedom isn't squelched.
Threesome meter: ****
Three-way challenge: emotional messiness

Pisces (February 20–March 20)
Hopelessly romantic, Pisces seeks deep emotional connections. Pisces tends to live in a fantasy world, where perfect love reigns supreme. Sparked by other people's energy, Pisces may feel energized in a threesome.
Threesome meter: ****
Three-way challenge: fantasy that there's only one prince charming

Capricorn (December 22–January 19)
Seeking security, commitment, and loyalty, Capricorn prefers fidelity and monogamy. Short-term three-way exploration may suit them, but anything more involved is probably off the table.
Threesome meter: *
Three-way challenge: attachment to monogamy

Sagittarius (November 22–December 21)
Gregarious, optimistic, and spontaneous, Sagittarius often fails to deliver when it comes to follow-through and long-term commitment. Threesomes may fulfill their need for adventure, hot sex, and freedom. Plus, three-ways might stave off Sagitarrius's major turn-offs—boredom and feeling trapped.
Threesome meter: ****
Three-way challenge: the urge for a power struggle

Scorpio (October 24–November 21)
Scorpio seeks hot sex, power, and loyalty. They're extremely jealous and possessive. Threesomes are unlikely to lure Scorpio, unless two doting submissives appear.
Threesome meter: **
Three-way challenge: jealousy and possessiveness

Libra (September 23–October 23)
Libra seeks harmonious relationships, lasting unions, and allurement. A threesome could be a delicious short-term adventure.
Threesome meter: ***
Three-way challenge: insecurities

Virgo (August 23–September 22)
Capable of being fulfilled by monogamy, Virgo seeks sensuality and long-term companionship. While threesome

flings may be enticing, Virgo may be too conventional for long-term triads.
Threesome meter: **
Three-way challenge: traditional mind-set

Leo (July 23–August 22)
Leo seeks excitement and security. Loyal at heart, they're inclined to stick with relationships, but may enjoy playing with other partners. Leo may welcome threesome flings with a long-term partner and a mysterious stranger.
Threesome meter: ***
Three-way challenge: self-centeredness

Aries (March 21–April 19)
Aries is energetic and dynamic with a strong love of adventure. Threesomes may be ideal for fun-loving Aries.
Threesome meter: ****
Three-way challenge: competitiveness

Taurus (April 20–May 21)
Likely to try a threesome with trusted friends, Taurus is sensual and seductive with a streak of jealousy and possessiveness. Personal-growth-oriented Taurus could use a threesome to boost inner security and overcome possessiveness.
Threesome meter: **
Three-way challenge: possessiveness and jealousy

Fire Signs (Aries, Leo, Sagittarius)

Fire seeks spontaneity, stimulation, freedom, and adventure. Fire's forte: one-night stands and fleeting lust. Marriage and long-term commitment may be a challenge.

Seduction tip: flattery, fun, and humor.

Fire^3: an intense, all-consuming, passionate roller-coaster relationship fueled by megahot sex.

Best three-way match: air.

Worst three-way match: earth, water.

Earth Signs (Taurus, Virgo, Capricorn)

Pragmatic and sense-oriented, earth seeks security and long-lasting connections. Biggest turn-on: dependable, long-term connections.

Seduction tip: sensual delights (i.e., food, wine, and candles).

Earth^3: a harmonious, lasting, and sensual connection.

Best three-way match: water.

Worst three-way match: air, fire.

Air Signs (Gemini, Libra, Aquarius)

The intellectual element that thrives on the world of ideas, air needs people to bounce ideas off . For air signs, love is a cerebral activity.

Biggest turn-ons: words, ideas, and inquisitiveness.

Biggest turn-offs: routine, lack of curiosity.

Air^3: a relationship with lots of cerebral sparks.

Best three-way match: fire.

Worst three-way match: water, earth.

Water Signs (Cancer, Scorpio, Pisces)

Water is the emotional element and wants to share emotions with others.

Biggest turn-on: emotional closeness. Water doles out sympathy and comfort.

Water^3: an empathetic and lasting relationship.

Best three-way match: earth.

Worst three-way match: fire, air.

Gemini (May 22–June 20)
A charming, entertaining lover, Gemini loves excitement and flirting. Since Gemini loves being the center of attention, threesomes may work best when Gemini joins a couple.
Threesome meter: ****
Three-way challenge: sharing the attention

Cancer (June 21–July 22)
Family-oriented Cancer probably considers monogamy the only way of life. Cancer is open to three-ways for sexual stimulation and extra cuddling but unlikely to want a long-term triad.
Threesome meter: **
Three-way challenge: attachment to security

Now that you've got a vision of your ideal three-way lovers, read the next section for the scoop on honing your three-way pickup mojo.

The Worst Thing About Threesomes: They're Too Hard to Set Up

Threesomes are lamer than doing cheap coke with your parents at a Linkin Park concert, in the rain, on your period, with a really itchy rash, during a breakup, in broken sandals. The question is: Why is something you looked forward to your whole entire adolescence so shitty?

—*Vice* magazine

GETTING YOUR THREE-WAY GAME ON: SEDUCTION 101

Three-way seduction requires more savvy, confidence, and technique than a one-on-one pickup. Threesomes usually form from a couple plus one, rather than three singles. And seduction strategy varies depending on whether your flying solo or hunting tandem. While single bi women have the pick of the litter in the threesome market, couples need more finesse to seduce a third. So before you rip off your leather vest and stammer a threesome request to a bombshell at a bar, arm yourself with some basic rules of the game. Below you'll find the nuts and bolts of priming your three-way mojo, seducing your new trio flame into the sack and special tips for tandem and solo hunting.

Sleaze Factor Warning: These three-way seduction strategies are intended to be used only with sensitivity, honest communication, and respect for boundaries. When inappropriately applied, these techniques may backfire, causing severe injury or death.

Classic Threesome Cockblock #1: Insecurity

Feeling insecure about your appearance or sexual prowess is a surefire way to flush a five-star threesome. So, know you're fabulous and strut your stuff.

Step 1. Get ready

So, you and your girlfriend are revving up to find a foxy third. Before you set foot in the pickup venue, tune up your confidence, body language, and style:

- **Up your confidence.** Attempting a three-way pickup opens you up to being called a pervy creep by the square community. Sure, some of your trio love interests may be too vanilla to try a three-way (sad, but true) and you'll likely face some rejection. But, you've got to be willing to take the risk or your chances are zilch. Being a wallflower might work occasionally for duo pickups, but it never works for three-way pickup—you've got to muster a shred of confidence and chutzpah to swing a three-way. Even at smut-loving venues such as swingers' clubs and parties, it can be intimidating to approach strangers. Be confident. Know that three-ways are the most common sexual fantasy, and it's totally cool to have three-way dreams. Don't let the fear of rejection stop you.

- **Use your body.** Seduction experts say 93 percent of the pickup is about body language rather than what you actually say. Make eye contact. You'd be surprised how far eye contact goes. If you meet someone fetching, start by making eye contact and holding it. Don't fidget. Fidgeting stinks of low self-confidence. And, smile, smile, smile.

- **Peacock.** Wear something outrageous or gaudy—anything that's a good conversation starter. Consider your orange velour jumpsuit a three-way pickup essential. Wearing something eye-catching is an ideal way to give people a way to start a conversation with you, and it also makes you look superconfident. Superconfident equals sexy.

Step 2. Open your mouth

Okay, so you and your girlfriend walk into a bar and you spot a gorgeous brunette laughing with her friends. Your girlfriend grins. She's mesmerized. So are you. So, what next?

- **Approach immediately**. You're cool and confident, so instead of hiding in the corner and waiting to divine a witty opening line, approach your target immediately. Don't wait more than three seconds before approaching. That leaves too much time to get psyched up and fink out.

- **Use an opener.** Some pickup artists swear by canned lines, others prefer to wing it. So experiment, be playful, and be brave. Openers range from direct threesome requests to disarming approaches that trick the target into feeling like a platonic friend (rather than

Tandem-Hunting Women: Three Approaches

Approach 1: Woman-to-woman

At venues with at least a partially straight crowd, women can approach other women posing as innocent pals, rather than three-way hunters on the prowl. Compliment her shoes or tattoo. Just start a conversation. Ask about her and show an interest. Direct openers also work for chick-on-chick pickup: hand her your number and say, "My boyfriend and I think you're gorgeous, so if you wanna make out sometime give us a call."

Approach 2: Guy-to-gal

Guys can approach a target solo. Use an indirect or a direct opener. "My girlfriend loves this place. Have you

a hunted sex object). Disarming openers are conversation starters about something seemingly innocuous. They work well with couples tandem-hunting a third, because most singles won't immediately assume a couple's hitting on them.

Step 3. Test your target's tri-curiosity and develop a connection

Okay, you survived the opener and your target is still talking to you. Now, it's time to take the connection a little deeper. Find out if the target meets your personal three-way standards and measure your target's tri-curiosity. Watch for signs of super squaredom. If your target's three-way interest seems to be nonexistent, don't heard the bizarre history of it?" Since you've mentioned your girlfriend, your target probably considers you an innocuous friendly guy and lets her guard down. Be charming. Then, your girlfriend appears and says, "Goodness, my boyfriend has fabulous taste in women."

Approach 3: The joint approach
Couples can approach single women together using direct openers like: "I'm Annie and this is Todd. We think you're beautiful. Do you want to come back to our place?" Or, try indirect, disarming openers like: "My girlfriend wants to name our new ferret after a 1990s game show, any ideas?"

waste your time. Exit and proceed to the next prospective three-way lovers. Here are some strategies for learning more about your target:

- **Games and gimmicks.** Some pickup artists use a range of gimmicks like tarot cards, magic tricks, runes, palm reading, or other psychological games. While these games border on smarmy, they work well as openers or to learn more about your target. And they work for testing your target's tricuriosity.

- **Be curious.** "Inner game"–based seduction artists say pickup is all about sincerity and genuine curiosity about someone. These experts keep a clear vision of what they want in lovers and use the first conversations as a discovery period to find out if there's potential for an interesting connection, rather than fishing for a one-night stand. Try to learn about the person by asking personal questions instead of generic questions. Shoot for questions like, "What are your hopes and dreams?" or "What's your happiest memory from this past week?" Then try broaching the threesome topic. Mention an article you read about open relationships. Mention that you're in an ethical open relationship. Mention that you're bisexual. See how the target responds.

The Cube

An old standard used by pickup artists. It hooks the target, builds a connection, and quickly gauges tri-curiosity. Here's the basic design:

> Have you ever done the cube? I'll ask some questions and when you've answered them, I'll know everything about you. Imagine a landscape. In the landscape there's a cube. Notice its size, color. What's it made of? Where is it? Next imagine a ladder. Notice where it is in relation to the cube. How big is it? What's it made of? Next you see flowers. How many are there? What color? What do they look like? Next, there's a horse. Describe it. Finally, there's a storm. Where is it? What's it doing?

• **Watch for tri-curiosity clues.** You've got to be able to identify who's open to a threesome, so you don't pass up an opportunity that's unfolding right before your eyes. We've all probably done that, and when it comes to threesomes, you've got to be extra tuned-in to pick up clues. Since threesomes are still closeted for the most part, many tri-curious people aren't sure if they're really get hit on by couples. Many tri-curious people say they never know if they're actually being propositioned by couples. So, stop assuming everyone is monogamous and watch for clues.

Cube: Self
Ladder: Aspirations or family or coworkers
Flowers: Friends
Horse: Ideal lover
Storm: Your life challenges

Then just make shit up—give obvious whacked-out answers for humor or pop psychology responses such as, "The cube is red, which means you're passionate." The cube can be used to determine whether the target's tri-curious. Describe the target as sexually adventurous, unconventional, or free-spirited. See how the target responds. Use the cube to deepen the connection and to learn more about the person. It beats asking, "So, what do you do for a living?"

She's Probably Tri-Curious If . . .

During a game of Truth or Dare she asks if you've ever been in a threesome.

She bites your neck and slaps your boyfriend's ass.

She squeezes between you and your lover on the dance floor.

She tells you she finds you and your boyfriend hot.

I can be a total dolt. One night my boyfriend and I were up all night with this blue-eyed hottie we met at a party. She was flirting with both of us. Even though her flirting got progressively more aggressive, I still didn't pick up on the fact that she wanted to have a threesome with us. Finally, she made it crystal clear by asking me: "If you could touch any vagina in the world right now, including mine, whose would you touch? Are you attracted to me?" So I kissed her.

—Gloria, 29

Step 4. Taking three-way seduction to the next level

Okay, your target is witty, intriguing, and sexy, and seems to be open to a threesome. Proceed to the next stages of the pickup: moving seduction to the next level.

- **Enjoy the flirting.** There are so many ways to flirt these days. Text messaging. Hair flipping. Double entendres. Where to begin? Instead of being goal-oriented about your threesome, enjoy the three-way flirting process. The buildup can be exquisitely titillating, especially if you're playing with a tri-virgin. Draw them in, make them wonder. Plus, the sex might be even hotter after a drawn-out courting process. (Even if you and your lover go home without a third, the flirting might prime you both for smokin' duo sex with three-way dirty talk.)

Classic Threesome Cockblock #2: Pushy Guys

A guy trying to bag two chicks to validate his ego is a surefire threesome repellant. And watching a guy pester his girlfriend into it isn't pretty, either. This common flub short-circuits potential threesomes. So lay low, guys.

- **Guys, play it cool.** Even if three-ways are your raison d'etre, don't be desperate. Overly eager tri-curious guys are a major three-way cockblock. Lower your trio-desperation by having personal standards about who you'll have threesomes with and by knowing that the universe will offer you threesomes when you're ready (just say om). If you've been chatting up a chick and you notice that her eyes are darting around the room, she keeps yawning and checking her watch, it's probably not the best time to tell her you'd like to see her tongue in your girlfriend's pussy. Desperation is always ugly, but exponentially so in threesome situations. Have some self-respect. If your target doesn't budge, move on. Don't chase. Give out your number, but don't ask for theirs.

- **Teasing and negs.** Negs are light jabs or teasing. Pickup artists develop negging skills, which they say work especially well on uber-bombshells, who are used to getting drooled over by hordes of horny men. It's a strategy for reeling in targets who are "out of your league" by bringing them down a notch through light teasing, instead of flattery, which they're used to and (often) sick of. Don't spark your target's deep insecurities (telling her she's got a hideous honker nose probably won't land her in the sack), but teasing her gently about her shirt might do the trick. The same approach works for handsome men, who are used to women melting at the mere sight of them. The bottom line: everyone likes a bit of a chase.

- **Move seduction to the next phase.** Directing the chemistry toward a threesome requires a delicate balance of leading and allowing—being overly pushy or aggressive is a massive turn-off, but if your target doesn't know clearly that you're interested in a threesome, they can't accept the offer. So lead the seduction gently. Take the initiative, rather than simply waiting for things to happen. And, make sure to physically escalate the seduction as soon as possible by touching your target on a neutral body part (such as the arm or wrist). Bring your target's attention to physical senses. Another way to escalate sexual tension is to create sexual barriers. This can be done various ways (such as, "I'd love to watch you two kiss, but the crowd in here wouldn't be able to take it.") Sexual barriers heighten the anticipation and get three-way juices flowing.

- **Establish the critical three-way link.** Threesomes require a connection between the two people in the same role. In other words, when straight couples seduce single women, the woman in the couple needs to establish a sparkly, noncompetitive dynamic with the single woman. If that link doesn't work, the threesome's probably a bust. Generally, the critical link needs to be established between the new person and the member of the couple most likely to have friction with the new person. Sometimes the critical link needs to be established between the new person and the shier, more reluctant member of the couple. Sniff out which critical link needs to be established and go for it.

Threesome Rule of Etiquette

Foot dragger's choice. One member of the couple is probably less enthusiastic or more insecure about a threesome; the shier person sets the pace and decides when, where, and who.

Step 5: Sealing the deal: the place, the mood, and the moves

There are various ways to bring a new flame back to your nest for a three-way. Try asking, "Do you want to come home with us?" Others suggest making an excuse to stop by your place. Experienced threesome seduction artists insist that setting the mood is key. When you're hosting, make your living room cozy and sensual. Hot tubs help. Then test these three-way starters:

- **The direct route.** Couples seducing a third will find it's much easier to get a three-way started if the woman takes the lead. Here are some ways she can get the three-way rolling:

> Try author Jen Sincero's favorite line for girl-on-girl pickups: "Do you want to make out?" It's simple, direct, playful, and who could resist?

Invite the third to make out with your partner: "Wow. I'd love to watch you kiss my boyfriend."

Ask the third, "Have you ever thought about having a threesome? Have you ever kissed a man/woman? Want to try? Have you ever tried a three-way french kiss?"

Mention that you've just read this fabulous book on threesomes and that you'd like to try one. Then ask, "Are you up for it?"

- **Bait and switch.** Tell your two hotties that you don't want to do anything sexual with them, but you'd love to just cuddle with them. Cuddling quickly leads to snuggling, snuggling turns into fondling, fondling turns into sucking, sucking turns into fucking. And, snap! Three-way booty bliss.

- **The clothing swap.** Costume changes are one way to get a three-way started. I've heard female seduction whizzes jump-start threesomes with: "Can I try on your bikini top?" Or ask your guests to try on your pink tennis skirt or leopard-print bustier. Clothing removal tends to move things in the right direction.

- **Dual-induction massage.** A pickup artist special, this technique involves telling your potential three-way playmates that receiving a massage from two people simultaneously creates a sensation overload that induces a deep, trancelike state. Then ask who wants to test it first. Ask the other masseuse to mirror your moves. Start with benign areas like the shoulders and back, then move toward the neck. Try running your lips over her neck and watch the other masseuse copy your moves. (This works best when a woman suggests it.)

- **Drinking games.** I Never, Spin the Bottle, and Truth or Dare. These games worked in seventh grade and they still work. When someone recommends these juvenile games, don't snub them. Consider the suggestion an indicator of interest—so if you're interested, just follow the simple sex-directed drinking-game script. Truth or Dare: ask only truth questions for the first three rounds. And, naturally, the questions should be sexual. Dares should be flirty, too (i.e., "I dare Johnny to unbuckle Karen's belt with his teeth.") It works every time. I Never works like this: Move in a circle; make a statement such as, "I've never been to Alaska or I've never been in a threesome," and whoever has been in the situation has to drink. Don't go off-script here or take things too deep—keep it light, flirty, and sexual. Asking about someone's relationship with her deceased mother or her sister's drug addiction is not a quick route into anyone's panties. (I've cockblocked beautiful threesome offers by accidentally asking the wrong question. I've also landed several yummy threesomes from drinking games.) Alternate between alcoholic drinks and energy drinks, to keep everyone sober enough to enjoy it.

- **Write a book on threesomes.** When people hear, they'll be pounding your door down to get in on the action.

- **Booze and drugs.** Booze can help lower inhibitions. But loads of potentially steamy three-ways misfire because someone gets too drunk or high to fuck. So if you use booze or drugs to lubricate your threesome, consider staying sober enough to get it on and enjoy it. And, limit the amount of liquor you serve your guests. Serve energy drinks to keep everyone perky.

Classic Threesome Cockblock #3: Over-Boozing

Over-boozing is one of the most common causes of threesome failure. Puking and passing out isn't sexy. Plus, guys often can't perform with too much booze in the blood.

Tequila Shots for Three

Put a lime in your mouth, salt your neck, then go in a circle with the tequila shot, neck-lick, lime-mouth kiss routine.

It's fine to rant about the dangers of illegal drugs, but the fact is, lots of people use them anyway. And, illegal drugs like ecstasy, marijuana, cocaine, ketamine, methamphetamine, and other designer concoctions are tried and true threesome starters. Ecstasy is a popular three-way catalyst because it heightens physical sensations and creates a serotonin surge strong enough to make kissing a cocker spaniel seem like a sexy idea. A word of caution: don't be the creepy drug pusher. If you're using recreational drugs and sharing them with others, make sure everyone involved knows the risks. While occasional ecstasy use probably won't kill you, drug cocktails can do you in for sure (even mixing illegal drugs with certain over-the-counter medications), so it's wisest to get the facts if you're going to partake. Plus, ecstasy can lead to depression, cocaine can be addictive, and meth can rot your brain at record speed, so research the side effects before deciding whether it's worth it to pop an illegal three-way inducer. Plus, guys on ecstasy (and other drugs) may have a difficult time getting it up. (Users say their best E-induced threesomes happened when the guy didn't take any or when the ecstasy started wearing off—while the inhibitions were still down, serotonin was still pulsing through the system, sensations were magnified, and the sun was rising.) (For risk assessment information on illegal drug use, check out: www.dancesafe.org, a nonprofit organization that promotes health and safety for recreational drug users.)

What I've regretted most about some of my threesomes is that I was too drunk and high to appreciate them. I don't regret doing them, I just regret being too messed up to remember and feel everything.

—Charles, 37

I was working in another city with these two beautiful women. They had been friends for years and they decided to take E one night. I declined the E. Next thing I knew, they were 69ing each other. And they invited me to join them. Ecstasy is the perfect three-way gateway drug. It was an incredible night.

—David, 38

Tales From the Dark Side: Threesomes That Flopped

I set up a three-way with two ex-girlfriends. It was so planned and we were all really nervous. One girl drank too much and ended up vomiting. By the time we actually started messing around, it was three AM, and I was exhausted. It was just too hard to maneuver.

—Rick, 25

> When I finally got a threesome going, I was too drunk to get it up. That blew. The chicks just went crazy on each other, and I was humiliated.
>
> —Jim, 22

TIPS FOR SEDUCING COUPLES, SINGLE WOMEN, SINGLE MEN, FRIENDS, AND STRANGERS

Tandem-hunting women

Couples on the prowl need teamwork. Generally, it works best when the man knows how to play it cool and give the women space to connect. Often tri-curious people decline three-way offers because the guy appeared to be pushing the three-way agenda too hard. Teamwork is key: the guy can lead (very subtly), by suggesting they all go to another fabulous bar across the street, but he needs to know how to stay in the background and let the women develop chemistry. The two women need to have sexual chemistry, or at least friendly, noncompetitive playfulness. In general, single women won't join couples unless they get a clear invitation from the woman in the couple. Only the woman in the couple can make it clear that she's not jealous and that she's turned on by the idea of a threesome. To cinch the deal: the woman in the couple needs to make it crystal clear that she's excited about bringing this woman home. Without that, only shark single women will oblige, resulting in an imbalanced, competitive threesome. So even if the guy starts the seduction, the woman in the couple needs to actively move the seduction along. Leading seduction can be a challenge for women who are used to taking a more passive role in seduction, but it's essential for three-way pickup. The woman needs to give a direct indication that she's hot for the single woman (tell her she's sexy) to avoid winding up in the platonic-friend category.

I'm constantly seeing cute couples I'd love to join for a night. It's hard to tell if a couple is flirting with me, because it's not what I'd normally expect (hint: be direct and explicit if you're trying to pick up a third for your conjugal bed).

—Rachel Kramer Bussel, *The Village Voice,* 2006

I recommend that you let the primary girl draft in the second girl because it's very scary for them. The first thing that happens when you tell your girlfriend you want another girl is she says, "Oh, shit, I'm not enough." If I brought home a second girl and said, "Look, honey," that just doesn't work.

—Stephane Hemon, seduction guru

Tandem-hunting men

It's usually acceptable for courteous and respectful male-female couples to directly approach hot prospects at a gay bar. Seducing a straight or bi-curious guy requires more finesse. The pickup generally runs smoothest with a woman ringleader. If the woman in the couple knows that her boyfriend is bi-curious, she can try testing the prospective lover's sexual openness and orientation by asking him if he's ever made out with a guy. If he doesn't flip out or scream homophobic slurs, she can say, "It would be so hot to watch you kiss my boyfriend."

If the man in the couple has no interest in experimenting with another man, the female ringleader can put the moves on the guy they're targeting. She can flirt and kiss the target. Then she can say that she and her boyfriend would like to take him home, but it's smoothest (considering that many American guys are still so homophobic) if she directly indicates that the threesome will be all about her and there won't be any guy-on-guy action. It's critical that her boyfriend makes it clear that he's inviting the other guy to join them and doesn't have any hang-ups about sharing his girlfriend. (No one wants to get smutty with a couple unless both members are open to it). Her boyfriend can even say, "I'd love to watch my girlfriend suck your cock."

Singles hunting couples

Singles hunting couples need to consider whether both members of the couple are into a threesome. Unless both members of the couple are tri-curious and enthusiastic about you, steer clear. Any hint that one of them has been bullied into it should be a warning bell. And any indications that the couple doesn't have their own boundaries and communication down pat should send you running. If they're über-hotties, but you're not sure they swing it three-way style, drop some hints. Tell them about the amazing threesome you had once, or tell them you've always wanted to try one. Enjoy watching their reactions.

Singles on the prowl for couples should target the person in the couple most likely to feel competition, jealousy, or unpleasant friction. If you've got chemistry with that person, then the trio has potential. Pay attention: if one member of the couple is shooting lightning bolts at you, a three-way isn't going to happen (and if it does, it probably won't be pretty). Use your intuition to gauge where to place most of your emphasis during the seduction and pay attention to both parties. Single women, pay attention to the woman in the couple. Is she giving you a good vibe? Single men, pay attention to the man in the couple. Is he giving you a good vibe?

If they both seem interested or if you're unsure about what they have in mind, clarify your intentions. To find out if you're all on the same page, be upfront and honest about your desires. If you'd like to schtoop the guy while his girlfriend watches, but you're straight and you don't want to kiss his girlfriend, let them know. If you just want to make out with the woman, try saying, "I'd like to make out with your beautiful wife while you watch. Is that cool with you?" Whatever it is, be honest. Pretending you're interested in both of them sexually could lead to a sticky, unpleasant threesome, so it's smartest to be up front. And you might find that they're into the same thing.

If you sense that one person in the couple is less enthusiastic, ask directly for clarification and get everyone's approval before proceeding. Don't assume anything. Sometimes, it's okay to kiss one member of the couple, but not the other. Every couple has different rules. If you're not entirely sure what's okay and what isn't, just ask. If you're kissing some woman's hubby, but the whole time you're wondering if you're overstepping your boundaries, you're less likely to have a good time. So, before you molest someone's partner, get clearance from the proper authorities. Don't know how the husband feels about you licking his wife's nipple? Ask him directly. Don't know if it's cool with the girlfriend if you fuck her boyfriend with a strap-on? Ask her directly.

A Quiz for Singles: Ten Ways to Spot a Threesome-Friendly Couple

1. She doesn't fly into a jealous fit when he winks at a cocktail waitress.
2. He doesn't sulk when she smiles at the handsome bartender.

3. They seem to have hot sex.
4. He hasn't coerced her into having a threesome. She hasn't coerced him.
5. They've *both* been giving you the eye.
6. They've been together for at least four years.
7. You're attracted to *both* of them.
8. They seem confident and secure with their relationship.
9. They communicate clearly and honestly with each other.
10. They have washboard abs.

Give yourself 2 points for each correct answer. A score of 8 or above is a safe bet; 6 or below means it's iffy; 4 or below is a definite no (think *Fatal Attraction*).

CREATING A NO-MUSS, NO-FUSS THREESOME FLING WITH STRANGERS

If your three-way goal is sexual spice pure and simple, orchestrate a no-strings-attached threesome with strangers by defining clear boundaries. First, don't have a three-way on your home turf. Meet your three-way partners at a bar or restaurant, then shack up in a hotel room, instead of inviting anyone over to your pad. Start a separate e-mail account just for threesomes and don't give out your home phone number. Find your three-way playmates at swingers' parties and other erotic-oriented events, so there aren't any expectations that sex will ooze into a relationship. Plus, in a crowd of pervs, you won't feel like an ass directly asking for a no-strings-attached threesome. Another way to ensure an unemotional threesome fling is to pay for it. Experienced sex workers have seen perverts of all stripes and generally won't look at you like you're a pathetic sleaze for your three-way aspirations.

Seducing friends

Many threesomes are harvested from friendships. Being open about your pervy dreams with friends may open the doors for interesting threesome adventures. If friends know that you're open to three-ways, often they just happen. If it's still not happening and you want to pursue a friend, start by testing the waters with questions. Ask if they've ever been in a threesome or if they've ever wanted to. If your friend is looking at you like you're a total freak, stop barking up the wrong tree. If you're getting some positive responses, continue. Mention that you and your boyfriend have been talking about it, and you think she would be fun to try it with. Plenty of successful threesomes happen among friends and many start with conversations about it. If you're concerned about messy emotional entanglements with your friend, talk openly and honestly about your intentions and expectations. Communicate clearly about you and your partner's boundaries. If you're in a couple, you can tell your friend clearly: "We're just interested in having fun with another person, but we're not interested in anything that comes between us. We've also agreed that we can only play with you when we're together. If that works for you, cool." That way, it's all clear. Ask your friend about her expectations and be honest about whether you're willing to meet those expectations. A super-direct communication blitz may suck a little of the spontaneity out of three-way seduction, so, ultimately, you might need to inject some extra romance to get the ball rolling.

> My husband and I propositioned a friend to have a threesome with us. We discussed it in detail, she agreed with the caveat that she needed to be "seduced." Enter: strawberries, chocolate, champagne, and whispered sweet nothings. Suddenly, the pants were off.
>
> —Anna, 24

Or, option B: Your boyfriend tries to kiss your friend while you're in the next room. Shocked, your friend resists, "Ooh, I can't do that. Your girlfriend is my friend!" (That's a standard, respectful response from friends unfamiliar with the world of open relationships.) Then your boyfriend says, "No, no, no. It's totally fine with her. I promise. Here, let's go ask her directly." Then, he brings the friend over to you and asks, "Do you mind if I kiss her?" You say: "Are you kidding? I'd love to watch you two kiss!" Friends who are totally unfamiliar with ethical nonmonogamy may take time to digest this. So if your friend doesn't go for it right away, be patient. Let it percolate.

Tales from the Trenches: Three-Way Pickups That Worked

I was at a party and this couple started a drinking game called I Never. The premise: drink if you've been in this situation. It started with innocent questions, like "Have you ever been to Minnesota?" Then, she asked, "Have you ever had group sex?" (I drank). After the party, they invited me over for drinks. They lit candles, put on some jazz, poured the wine, and snuggled next to me on the couch. After several hours of putting the moves on, she finally invited me to join them in bed. They were so nervous that it was charming. I went for it and I'm glad I did!

—Lisa, 31

I'm a 100 percent straight guy. My girlfriend took me to a gay bar and this femme guy started hitting on me. My girlfriend said she thought it would be hot if I made out with him. So, he came back to our place, where he blew me while I went down on my girlfriend and, basically, serviced me royally. Then I fucked my girlfriend while he ate my ass. I came so hard. My girlfriend and I both want to do this again.

—Bob, 34

My boyfriend and I used to seduce women into threesomes. We found that the aftermath was too much of pain in the ass. Now, we just offer an ambiance of safety, decadence, and deviance. We're open about what we do and we wait for women to come to us. That way, the women we end up sleeping with are those who really want to do it and aren't going to freak out about it afterwards.

—Marne, 26

Troubleshooting: Eliminating the Fourth

One of the biggest threesome juggernauts: a fourth person. Often two couples are interested in threesomes. There are various ways to bypass (or surgically remove) a fourth. One solution: wait until one person is passed out drunk or at the office. If there's a high enough comfort level between the foursome, sometimes it's possible to directly negotiate a threesome exchange. (Another option: what's wrong with four? Maybe more is even merrier.) Or, at the least, the fourths can take turns watching and participating.

My friend and her husband were at my place for drinks. When her husband passed out, I had a nice little threesome with my friend and my boyfriend. She gives amazing blowjobs, so I wanted my boyfriend to experience that. It was sexy. She had an agreement with her husband and when he woke up the next day, he laughed and called asking why he hadn't gotten a thank-you-for-the-blowjob-from-my-wife card. He was totally fine with it.

—Danielle, 28

You're well on your way to becoming a three-way lothario; now, read the next section for the scoop on where to meet your dream three-way lovers.

SCENES TO SCOPE OUT: THE HOT SPOTS FOR THREE-WAY PICKUP

Ideally, everyone into three-ways would have a 3 tattooed on their foreheads. Since that isn't the case, you never know who'll be down for it until you try. That means you'll risk getting an ew-you're-a-perv glare. Remember that most people have had three-way fantasies even if they're unwilling to admit it at a cocktail party. Sex studies show that the majority of sexually active adults have at the very least fantasized about having sex with more than one person at a time. So let your trio flag fly.

Personally, I've found that often the most unlikely people are up for it. I met one couple at my most conservative friend's dinner party; they hit on me for hours, but I still couldn't actually believe it until they spelled it out with a formal invitation to join them in bed. So when you start watching for signs of tri-curiosity, you might find threesome potential everywhere. But, where do tri-curious people hang out?

If you're new to the three-way game, it's easiest to start in venues that draw an "open-minded" crowd—freaks, geeks, porn junkies, bohemians, rockers, and artists. Think: strip clubs, drag shows, and swingers' parties. Plus, if you go for people who are comfortable trisexuals, you're more likely to have a dazzling experience without as much turmoil and emotional processing. In general, polyamory events, personals, and Web sites tend to focus more on building long-term unconventional relationships, and lifestyle events/erotic parties tend to focus more on no-strings-attached sex (though lots of swingers become close friends with their sex buddies). The major bonus of getting down three-way style with swingers, polyamorous people, or online pickups is that your playmates already know the score. If they're in the scene, chances are they've already worked through their own hang-ups and they're ready to plunge in without needing a diatribe on the benefits of group sex. So whether you're seeking an emotional triad relationship or a threesome fling, below you'll find a list of the best venues for meeting your ideal three-way lovers.

As you venture into various threesome-friendly scenes, know that each scene has very different rules of behavior and bone up on each scene's etiquette in advance. When you get there, don't immediately start shamelessly fondling strangers or assume that everyone there will be willing to jump in the sack with you, just because they're at an "open-minded" event or "sex-positive" venue. Respect other people's boundaries and each event's rules of etiquette. Being openly tri-curious is fabulous, but aggressively trying to bag two chicks to pump up your ego is another thing. Be forewarned: many scenesters don't take kindly to frat-boy-style aggressiveness and unprompted ass groping. They'll eat you alive for that shit (and erotic parties will actually boot you from the event). The most basic rules to remember: don't be an asshole and get verbal consent *before* you touch.

Online

There are dozens of ads placed by straight couples seeking the mythical elusive "hot bi babe" in newspapers across the country. I've heard some (though limited) success stories on this front. Some three-way veterans swear by personal ads and online dating, others say you've got to weed through too many misses to hit the right chemistry. Craiglist is smut central, offering everything from SWM interested in watching couples have sex to "spiritual couples" seeking bisexual women to live with them and bear their children. There's something for everyone. Potential three-way playmates can also be contacted via Yahoo personals. E-mail someone you fancy about your threesome interest. If she's interested, take her on a date and see where it leads. One major perk: there's no need to be coy about your three-way interest—just be clear and direct about what you want, and whoever isn't into it gets weeded out.

Necessary Seduction Accouterments: saucy digital pics

Bi-Curious and a Little Nervous . . .

I am a relatively innocent white female, interested in a first-time experience with woman or couple. I have always found other women attractive, especially large breasts, and would like to have a one-time play date to explore my fantasies. I would like to play with a woman while her man watches or participates (minimally). I will not have intercourse with him, but will watch while they do. I'm new to this and a little nervous but willing to give it a shot!

—Personal ad, The Wild Side, *City Paper*

- **Online groups.** Whatever it is that floats your boat, you're likely to find an e-mail group for it online. There are also Yahoo polyamory and swinging groups from South Africa to New York City with support, events, matchmaking, and more. Even Boston has an active polyamory Yahoo group with more than two thousand members. The major perk of these online groups is that you can find an exact match for your own perverted tastes, which makes getting your freak on much easier. For example, there's a Yahoo e-mail group with hundreds of bisexual women in Southern California—most members are openly bisexual women who are married to men and date women on the side. The group hosts weekly events, gatherings, and meet-ups. The perks of the group: everyone on the list is openly bisexual, so sexual identity confusion is less likely and they won't scoff at "fence-sitters" or nonmonogamous types. There's a Yahoo group for just about everyone, so find one that suits your particular three-way itch.

- **Online three-way dating tips.** Don't prolong the e-mail exchange too long. Meet ASAP for a chemistry check. Since some people complain that craiglist personals are flooded with men posing as bisexual women, it's wise to talk on the phone before meeting to verify that your online match is who they say they are. When you meet an online hookup, leave your date's name and phone number with a friend. And never give an online date your home address before you meet them. But don't be totally paranoid.

- **Polyamory versus "lifestyle" matchmaking sites.** The major difference between polyamory and lifestyle personals is that polyamory personals focus on multiple

Personal-Ad Lingo

NSA: no strings attached

LTR: long-term relationship

HBB: hot bi babe (the elusive holy grail of threesomes, the most sought-after third wheel by tri-curious straight couples across the nation)

TG: transgender

The 411

www.craigslist.com

www.polymatchmaker.com

www.yahoo.com (personals)

www.nerve.com

www.AdultFriendFinder.com

www.backpage.com

www.lifestylelounge.com (a fee-based membership with member profiles across the nation, instant booty-call section, event listings, and more)

http://alt.com

www.yahoogroups.com (search polyamory, swingers, lifestyle, open relationships, etc.)

www.meetup.com

relationships, while lifestyle personals focus on booty calls. Polyamory matchmaking sites feature people seeking a smorgasbord of relationship types, from triad relationships to five-person group marriages. Explore each site and have a clear vision of what you're looking for before posting your bio.

- **Watch for the classic bait and switch.** Couples seeking single bi women for threesomes often get responses from a supposedly single woman, then surprise! She brings her boyfriend along to watch.

Polyamory clubs, meetings, and events

If you're looking for a one-night threesome, polyamory events aren't for you. Polyamorists tend to be more interested in developing romantic connections with sex partners. Polyamory groups host support groups, meetings, and parties all over the world. Register for a polyamory e-mail list to find out about local events. There's a strong "say what you mean" vibe at poly events, which might shock playful flirts new to the scene. Generally, poly folks can be a bit "processy" (talk about how you're feeling and how you feel about talking about how you're feeling ad nauseam). Though, attending a poly dinner is bound to hone your communication skills, challenge you to think about relationships in a new way, and offer helpful advice on threesome-related snafus (and you might even get some play).

Necessary Seduction Accouterments: clear, Direct communication style

The 411

www.polyamory.com

www.polyamory.org

www.nfnc.org (hosts an annual "Summer Camp" for polyamorous people)

www.PartnerPlayshop.org

www.lovemore.com

www.lovewithoutlimits.com

www.polyamorysociety.com

www.worldpolyamoryassociation.com

What Does Polyamory Have to Do with Three-Ways?

Polyamory is an umbrella term used to describe multiple romantic relationships happening concurrently. The difference between polyamory and old-fashioned cheating? Polyamorists don't lie, cheat, or steal to get booty. Polyamory relies on honest communication and consent from everyone involved. Those who identify as poly often say they consider relationships more important than sex. Self-identified poly people are less likely to roam the streets looking for one-night threesome flings and more likely to become involved in longer-term or emotionally involved triad relationships with friends or other poly people from meet-ups.

Geek central: Ren Faire, gaming, and science fiction conventions

There's major crossover between the sci-fi fandom and polyamory, owing partly to 1960s science fiction writer Robert Heinlein and his polyamory-promoting novels (such as *Strangers in a Strange Land*). Many sci-fi geeks love in triangles, quads, or open relationships of some form. And sci-fi conventions have hosted triad marriage ceremonies. If geeks make you hot, brush up on your Klingon.

Necessary Seduction Accouterments: Klingon dictionary

The 411

www.wordcon.org (an annual convention with a large population of polyamorous people and poly-related discussion panels)

www.scificonventions.com

www.renfaire.com.

www.sca.org (an international organization dedicated to researching and recreating pre-seventeenth-century European arts and crafts, includes many polyamorous members, and local clubs offer one route into the Ren Faire scene)

Art parties/events

Freaks notoriously frequent art openings and art-related parties. Historically, artists have tended to be more open to unconventional sexual expeditions and romances. Famous artist clans that indulged in nonmainstream sexuality include the 1920s Greenwich Village bohemian scene with its lesbian chic and the turn-of-the-century Bloomsbury artists (including Virginia Woolf) who embraced open marriage. Artists still tend to be more experimental when it comes to sex and love. Groups all over the world host off-the-hook counterculture art parties.

Necessary Seduction Accouterments: style

The 411

www.Tribe.net (check out groups such as "ethical sluts," "polyamory," and "fluid marriage")

www.GenArt.com (sign up for e-mail event announcements for hip art happenings)

www.oregoncountryfair.com

http://massiveburn.org (an organization promoting art and music events)

www.flavorpill.com (sign up for weekly e-mail event announcement with cultural happenings)

Most modern art museums in most cities also offer evening events for hipsters. Sign up for e-mail event announcements at your local museum.

Alternative lifestyle events: old-school swingers and the new modern

"The lifestyle" doesn't have a sexy image these days. It seems like a vestige of 1970s key parties and conjures images of pasty seniors getting sweaty together in shag-carpeted, Orange County clubhouses. While this cadre of swingers exists, there's a new generation of swingers now—they're young, hip, and drop-dead gorgeous. Instead of using the outdated "swinger" label, these hipsters call themselves "modern." And, "modern" parties are springing up all over the country and catering to everyone from conservative East Coast intellectuals to Seattle hipsters to Tinseltown celebrities. And this scene can be exclusive: top lifestyle parties are private, only admit partiers under age thirty-five, and require photos and bios in advance. One enthusiastic modern guy reports: "I thought there would be old, unattractive, uncool people at swingers' parties. That's just the image I always had of swingers. But, the first time I went, I couldn't believe it. They were amazingly beautiful, attractive people—and there wasn't an extra ten pounds of fat among all six hundred of them. I knew that it was for me."

VOCABULARY BUILDERS

Modern

The twenty-first-century version of swinging. Generally used to mean open-minded, free-thinking, and nonjudgmental, the term was coined by Naomi (the lioness), hipster queen of the A-list Hollywood lifestyle scene. "Modern" people aren't hung-up on monogamy.

Old-fashioned

The opposite of modern. Used to describe someone in a closed relationship and set on monogamy.

Alternative lifestyle parties are all very different, so if one doesn't work for you, don't snub the whole scene before trying another one. The scene is so diverse that it's hard to judge the whole scene based on a single event. Some lifestyle parties are homophobic when it comes to guy-on-guy action and, while girl-on-girl action is common, some bisexual women consider the girl-on-girl action too exhibitionist or performance oriented. Other lifestyle parties embrace all sexual orientations.

The new generation of moderns distinguish themselves from polyamorists, saying that their sexual playmates are "just for fun," while poly people tend to dive into relationships. Many moderns, however, develop long-term, intimate friendships with their fuck buddies. There's a huge range of options and preferences within the "modern" community—some couples prefer to date other couples (or singles) for months before getting frisky with them, others are up for a roll in the hay with hotties they've just met.

Lifestyle organizations host cocktail nights and late-night parties, where threesomes can be concocted in a night. And, studies show that 90 percent of swingers have participated in threesomes. One major bonus: squares have been weeded out, so no one's going to be miffed by a direct threesome request. If you're hesitant, try an off-site sex party or erotic party first, where modern people meet, flirt, and fondle. Then, when you're feeling friskier, try an on-site sex party (sometimes called a play party), where moderns actually get down to business at the party.

Lifestyle party etiquette 101. Most modern parties are unique drama-free, female-centered, safe spaces that invite smutty exploration. Women run the scene. Most lifestyle and erotic parties create an atmosphere where women feel comfortable exploring their naughty interests without getting lecherously hit on by men. Seasoned guys on the scene know how to lay low and follow the women's lead. Unlike most straight bars, men don't hit on women at modern parties. Women approach their targets, flirt, and initiate sexual contact. The best pickup line I've heard at a lifestyle party: "I was a lesbian for five years, I'm over that, but I'd like to lick your pussy and make you cum all night long." (Who wouldn't be charmed by those credentials?) Basically, the lifestyle motto can be summed up: "Men behave, women go wild." Single men aren't allowed into most modern parties, and one erotic play party club even requires single men to wear "badges" so they can be booted easily if they misbehave. General rules include: don't get too drunk, respect perversity in diverse forms, and don't aggressively cruise (unless you're a woman). Get permission and be willing to accept a no.

Necessary Seduction Accouterments: low-key attitude (for men) and pickup lines (for women)

The 411

www.Kinkysalon.com (a Bay-area club that hosts pansexual erotic play parties)

www.Tribe.net (join the kinkysalon tribe to find similar events)

www2.cakenyc.com (a community that throws female-oriented erotic parties)

www.lustparty.com (an exclusive lifestyle community in Los Angeles—members must be under thirty-five and submit photos and bios to be admitted)

www.Lifestylelounge.com (the major personals site for modern people, features dozens of lifestyle event listings across the nation)

www.nasca.com (an international swingers' association)

www.swingclubs.us (a source for swing clubs and events nationwide)

www.eros.com (an erotic-oriented Web site that lists lifestyle parties and events nationwide)

www.lifestyles-convention.com (hosts an annual megaconvention)

The 411

www.br.org (a Washington, DC-based SM club)

www.threshold.org (an education group and party host in Los Angeles)

www.soj.org (a San Francisco-based BDSM group)

Bondageball.com (fetish event listings)

www.paddlesnyc.com (hosts spanking parties in NYC)

Necessary Seduction Accouterments: latex jumpsuits

BDSM and other kink-friendly events

There are endless opportunities to get your freak on at BDSM parties and clubs that range from light costume fetish balls to hard-core "edge play" shindigs. I've seen an eighty-year-old pharmacist hung from the ceiling by flesh hooks in his back, an eighteen-year-old woman have her mouth sewn closed with medical sutchers, and other adrenaline boosting phenomenon in private SM clubs. Obviously, the crowd at these places tends to be open to a range of sexual experiences and three-ways are unlikely to ruffle any feathers. Most SM venues host orientations—a must for newbies.

Sex-shop classes

Many sex shops host classes on various topics from bondage to oral sex technique. Some even invite students to share cocktails and mingle after the class. Voilà—a shared interest in something pervy. Jen Sincero, author of the *Straight Girls' Guide to Sleeping with Chicks,* teaches classes at sex shops nationwide, and many of the women attending her classes have boyfriends/husbands and are looking to date women on the side or have threesomes. It's a perfect way to meet women up for threesomes. (Note: The class is for women only, so guys looking for two women are out of luck.)

Necessary Seduction Accouterments: vibrator batteries and edible undies

The 411

www.thepleasurechest.com

www.babeland.com

www.goodvibrations.com

Hippie events and pagan ceremonies

Follow the patchouli. Open-minded hippies are often well versed at following their hearts, and they're less likely to buy into suburban values. If tie-dye and tantra make you hot, seek out hippie-magnet venues such as clothing-optional resorts (though some emphasize they're "not for swingers"), tantric sex workshops, organic bean-sprout festivals, tofu workshop ceremonies, and yoga studios.

Necessary Seduction Accouterments: unshaven pits

The 411

www.harbinhotsprings.com (a Bay-area clothing-optional resort that hosts tantric workshops)

www.schooloftantra.com (a Hawaii-based school that hosts workshops and events year-round)

www.clubtantra.org

www.sexyspirits.com

www.clubtantra.com

www.caw.org (Church of All Worlds, the first pagan church founded in the United States—inspired by Robert Heinlein's sci-fi novels, which popularized the concept of group marriage)

www.nudistseek.com (lists nudist resorts all over the world—some are lifestyle friendly, others aren't)

www.circlesanctuary.org (Circle Sanctuary is a nonprofit featuring events related to nature, spirituality, paganism, and Wiccan ways.

www.paganet.org (lists pagan events nationwide)

Raves and dance clubs

Raves and high-energy dance clubs are hubs for drug-soaked masses (crowds are on the younger side). The scenes host various partiers from silicon-infused porn stars to young piercing-clad ravers to dread-sporting hoola-hoopers; many are sexually experimental. Venues range from five-thousand-person mega dance clubs to underground industrial warehouse raves. Again, it's key to know the etiquette for this crowd: ecstasy-bombed partiers will likely run shrieking from a smarmy vibe. Ecstasy causes a surge in serotonin, an overwhelming warm, fuzzy feeling, lowered inhibitions, and heightened physical sensations. Learn to cuddle properly, without being pushy, and triple sensory pleasure might bloom.

Necessary Seduction Accouterments: colorful costumes, fuzzy clothing, water bottles, flavored lip gloss, decent dance moves, and good vibes

The 411

Find out about local events through record store fliers.

www.tribe.net (local nightlife tribes)

www.loveparade.net (a massive dance event with more than 1.5 million visitors)

Straight bars and other venues frequented by squares

Hitting straight bars for cold three-way approaches is best left to seasoned three-way flirts. Until you've mastered scoring a three-way at a pagan love ceremony or a strip club, straight bars are likely to stump you. Of course, it all depends on how your three-way mojo works, and if it's in mint condition, a well-liquored crowd with some seductive music and dimly lit corners could be ideal for three-way pickup. Cardinal no-nos: desperation and three-way shame.

Necessary Seduction Accouterments: guts, confidence, and fabulous style

Gay bars

Male-female couples looking to snag a guy may have a relatively easy time ferreting out a hot gay or bi man at a gay bar. There's no need to perfect pickup strategy, just set your sights on what you want and go for it. One thirty-six-year-old gay man explained, "The nice thing about gay bars is you don't have to buy anyone flowers. You can just get together and have a good time." Feel free to be boldly direct about your sexual wishes—if the chemistry is there, you probably won't get a smack in the face for directly requesting a threesome. And plenty of gay men are up for playing the initiator for straighties.

Since much of gay male culture accepts open relationships to some extent, the threesome concept won't totally shock or baffle most men in gay bars. It's not uncommon for long-term, committed gay male relationships to adopt "don't ask, don't tell" policies, agreements that allow threesomes when both partners are present, or open relationships with limits on external play (oral sex with others might be okay, but intercourse might not). And gay male triads have been known to last successfully for decades—where all partners live together, share a bed, and share incomes. So couples picking up a guy from a gay bar will likely have an easier time swinging a threesome with minimal energy investment in helping the third "emotionally process" the situation.

And, M^3 threesomes are relatively easy to orchestrate with three singles at a gay bar. I've interviewed dozens of men who have enjoyed one-night threesomes with pickups from a gay bar. One gay writer said, "I never go out looking for a threesome, they generally just happen. I've had lots of them. They've all been with three single guys getting together, rather than a couple. I'm reluctant to join a couple unless I know them really well, because I don't know if they have things worked out or whatever." So, if there's three-way chemistry, just say, "We'd like to bring you home tonight."

I was at a party at a designer's loft, then I went back to my friend's place with him and his friend. Everyone was equally into each other. I was giving this cute guy a blowjob and getting fucked from behind at the same time. It was perfect. It was great gay sex. Everyone got off and it didn't mean anything. We ate breakfast and watched a movie the next day. No drama. No complications.

—Greg, 33

Necessary Seduction Accouterments: decent grooming

Lesbian bars

Whether you're scouting a hip, West Hollywood ultra-femme scene right out of *The L Word* or a butch dive bar in Buffalo, straight couples might not have an easy time finding a third in the lesbian bar scene. Bisexual women aren't always welcomed with open arms and when they are accepted, it's usually when they've left their boys at home. On the other hand, some lesbian couples indulge in boy toys for a night. Single men lurking about lesbian bars alone probably won't be so welcome, unless they're extremely respectful and courteous. Those lucky enough to find openly bisexual woman hanging at the dyke bar might have an ideal combo. Bisexual women who've successfully picked up lesbians for threesomes say it works best when the woman goes out hunting alone, but it's generally wise to let the pickup know that there's a guy waiting back at home.

Necessary Seduction Accouterments: strong hands

Vacation

If you're too timid to try a three-way in your hometown, take a vacation. Just getting away from your daily scene can help free up your freaky side. (Plus, you'll never have to see your three-way playmates again). Vacationers tend to let their guard down and explore sexual behaviors they're reluctant to try at home. Find other travelers and get your three-way groove on. The best threesome vacation spots feature an active dance club scene, outdoor raves (such as Thailand's infamous full moon parties), and sensual delights such as good food, wine, and massage. These spots have been cited for top-notch party scenes and foster the best environments for sexual exploration.

The 411

Best Three-Way Vacation Spots

Ibiza

Bali

College spring-break spots (Daytona Beach and Cancun)

San Francisco

Berlin

Goa, India

Thailand

London

Mykonos, Greece

Vancouver

South Beach, Florida

Kauai

Necessary Seduction Accouterments: string bikini and a strawberry daiquiri

Strip clubs and burlesque shows

Strips clubs generally attract a relatively open-minded crowd and three-way veterans report success picking up threesome playmates in these spots. Modern burlesque shows, which have become trendy in the past few years, are also solid three-way pickup venues.

Necessary Seduction Accouterments: fishnet stockings

The 411

www.sweetandnastyburlesque.com

www.velvethammerburlesque.com

suicidegirls.com (a touring burlesque show featuring punk-style dancers complete with tatts and piercings)

www.starshineburlesque.com

Hire a pro

Hiring a sex worker is one way to get comfortable with a third party without worrying too much about jealousy. One woman said, "I hired a stripper to be in a threesome with me and my boyfriend. She didn't do much, she was really just there to look pretty. I got really turned on watching her kiss my boyfriend. There's a fine line between jealousy and getting turned on. I guess she just wasn't a threat, so I didn't have any jealousy. It worked out perfectly." One advantage of hiring a professional is that a pro can help you feel more relaxed about the whole thing. Based on interviews with sex workers who have been hired by couples, here's the skinny on hiring a three-way playmate:

1. Figure out what you want. Do you want someone to come over and dance for you? Do you want someone to lick your wife's pussy? Do you want someone to massage you both? If you want someone to just dance for you and your hubby without having any physical contact, hire a stripper for a strip-club style show. If you're interested in getting more intimate, but maybe not scoring the whole caboodle, consider hiring a stripper or sensual masseuse. If it's penetration you're after, seek out an escort.

2. Go online. Search the categories: sensual massage, escorts, and dancers/strippers. Read the bios and look at photos. If tantric sex floats your boat, seek out a "dakini" (tantric sex priestess). Some will perform "sacred spot" massage (meaning they'll root around for your G-spot and show your lover how to find it).

VOCABULARY BUILDER

GFE

(Girlfriend Experience)

Dancers/escorts who include "GFE" in their ads pride

themselves on building connections with clients, rather than the wam-bam-thank-you-mam variety service.

3. Make the calls. Sure, it's important to select someone whose photo gets you going, but it's even more important to have a good conversation with her on the phone. Don't book based on photos alone. You may have to call several people before you reach the right one. Tell her you've never done this before and you're interested in a couple's show. Ask if she's into women (or if you're hiring a male dancer, if he's into men). Use your time on the phone to get a vibe reading of the person. If you get the sense that she's a genuine, nice, smart person, and she seems excited about it, that's a good sign. Don't explicitly negotiate sex acts over the phone. Most escorts won't feel comfortable discussing details about sex over the phone, since that's one way to land your butt in jail. Strippers, however, are more likely to talk about details on the phone. Generally, it's wisest to use some code words, especially when you're talking to escorts (*full service:* intercourse, *greek style:* anal sex). If you know exactly what you're looking for, ask by alluding to it. It's okay to ask: "Are you comfortable using toys?" but don't ask: "Are you okay with fucking my wife with a double-ended dildo?" Ask if he or she's comfortable "getting intimate with couples" or "are you comfortable getting interactive with my girlfriend"? (Some dancers will only perform for couples without having any physical contact; others will kiss, lick, and more.) Ask and she'll give you a clue about whether physical contact is off-limits.

> I do lots of shows for couples when I kiss the woman's nipples while she's having sex with her husband. Most of us get excited to do couples' shows. It means we get to do something out of the ordinary and it's exciting to see two people really in love spicing up their sex lives. My advice is to find a stripper who says, "I love doing couples' shows."
>
> —Erotic dancer, Seattle

4. Plan in advance. Don't wait until Saturday to decide you want to hire a stripper that night. Book in advance and it's best not to schedule on a Friday or Saturday night. If she's busy with parties (which pay big), she's likely to be in a rush, and that can spoil the mood. If you insist on a weekend booking, schedule a late Friday night (ask if you're her last show for the night) or a Sunday evening. Ask what works best with her schedule so she can take her time. Reserve a few hours. It's just as important to have time to sit, talk, and sip wine together before jumping into the sexual play. If you're unsure about whether you've hired the right person and don't want to commit to more than one hour, have enough cash on hand to ask for an additional hour if you're having a good time and want to spend more time together.

5. Welcome brigade. Pay up first. When she arrives, hand her the cash (and a tip doesn't hurt). That way, she'll be relaxed during the show, and if you've paid her well, she's more likely to feel free to go further. Don't negotiate or offer tips during sexual acts—that's illegal and might make her feel uncomfortable. If you booked an hour, when the hour is up and you'd like her to stay longer, tell her you're having a great time and you'd love for her to stay for another hour if she's into it. If she agrees, pay her for another hour. (Some dancers will offer a discount on the second hour—it's kosher to ask about this over the phone in advance). When you meet in person, state your boundaries explicitly. Tell her what you're interested in and what your limits are. Then, sit back, spend some time chatting, and see where it leads.

6. Mind your manners. Always ask permission before you touch. Don't just reach out and touch the stripper's pussy just because you feel like it. Err on the side of caution, by asking. "Are you comfortable with me licking your nipples? Would you be comfortable watching us have sex now?" Strippers say they love it when clients ask, and it avoids awkward situations. Understand that female dancers will often be more permissive with other women than with men. So just because your wife can touch the stripper's pink doesn't mean she'll feel comfortable with you doing it. Just ask. And don't try to get her to change her mind or push her boundaries if she says no. Persistence can be ugly. Plus, if you mind your manners, she might offer some unexpected treats.

7. Be flexible. Have low expectations, especially if you've hired a stripper as a surprise for your lover. Surprises can be exhilarating, but, if you've never talked about this with your partner, don't expect them to react with glee. Even if you've discussed the fantasy of bringing in a third, the surprise could make your lover shy. So keep an open mind.

A good stripper knows something about psychology and will generally take the shier person's lead. If a guy hires me as a surprise for his girlfriend, I take it really slowly. Maybe we'll touch her a little. Maybe that's all we'll do that day, but I'm not going to walk in there and pressure her to fuck me with a double-ended dildo. Even when a girlfriend hires me as a surprise for her boyfriend, she needs to be prepared to modify her original expectations. Sometimes the guy might have so much anxiety about having another person in the room that he can't get an erection or he's just weirded out by it, even though he's been fantasizing about it for decades. Just be flexible and be prepared to take it slow.

—Erotic dancer, NYC

Necessary Seduction Accouterments: a fat wad of cash and a polite attitude

The 411

www.eros.com (a nationwide online directory listing thousands of escorts, dancers, and fetishists of all sorts to stir your burning three-way passion)

www.Myredbook.com (a Bay-area directory for escorts, dancers, and more)

www.cityvibe.com

www.theeroticreview.com (a fee-based site that offers detailed reviews of erotic dancers and escorts)

THREE-WAY SEDUCTION EXERCISES

1. Make a list of five qualities you want in a threesome playmate. Create your own boundaries. Who do you consider off limits and why? Make a list of prospective threesome playmates. Talk to your partner. Do you both agree?

2. Decipher your own three-way fantasies. Are you itching for same-sex experimentation? Or are you hankering to watch or be watched? Are you interested in playing with an openly bisexual or gay playmate? Or would a straight playmate work better for you? Are you interested in no-strings-attached three-way sex or three-way intimacy? Talk to your partner: express your threesome interests and listen to your partner talk about his.

3. Couples considering a friend for a threesome: create a vision with limits ahead of time. Do you want a regular three-way fuck buddy? Will it be okay for each of you to sleep with her independently afterward? How close do you want to bring that friend into your life? Are you both willing to sever ties with the friend if the trio gets too intense or if either of you feel your relationship is being threatened?

4. Assess your potential third. How do you feel physically after spending time with a potential third? Your own physical response can be an indicator of whether the third is a healthy match for you and your partner. If you feel drained every time, this third might not work best for you.

5. Test five different openers on strangers.

CHAPTER 4

THREE CAN BE A CROWD: STRATEGIES FOR NAVIGATING FREAK-OUTS, JEALOUSY, AND GENERAL MESSINESS

My girlfriend of six years started kissing this girl we brought back to our hotel room. I watched them go at it. Then my girlfriend lifted her skirt and pointed her ass towards me. My dick started going limp because I was super nervous, so I started going down on my girl. She loved it. My girl started kissing the other girl's tits and banging her, next my girl hinted at me to bang the other girl. I hesitated and looked at my girl, trying to figure out what she wanted, then my girlfriend grabbed my hand and directed my fingers into the other girl's pussy. My girl got on top of me

> and started riding me with my legs off the bed and the other girl sat on my face. So I licked her pussy. Suddenly my girl got off me and started crying. I asked her why. She wouldn't say anything and just continued to make out with the girl. We finished up about twenty minutes later and said good-bye to the other girl. As soon as the door closed, my girl gave me this weird look. I have never heard the end of it *ever.* My girl said it was a test and I failed, and if I loved her I never would have done that.
>
> —Andre, 31

Sure, it's tempting to jump into three-way sexcapades without considering the consequences, but you could wind up with an emotional shit-storm rough enough to obliterate your self-esteem and spoil your relationship. Punch-your-grandma-in-the-face threesome sex sans emotional fallout requires prep work and a big commitment to honest communication.

In order to make three-ways hot and fulfilling for everyone involved, you'll have to be willing to take an honest look at yourself and to do a lot of talking. Know that going from a traditional monogamous relationship to having a threesome will involve some growing pains—after all, it requires learning new skills and getting over a lifetime of social conditioning. Often threesome newbies discover intense insecurities and fears based on outdated beliefs about themselves, their partners, or relationships in general. So, enter your three-way ventures with a curious attitude about what you'll learn about yourself, instead of dashing back to safety as soon as you hit an emotionally uncomfortable pothole. This chapter gives you the lowdown on how to prepare for a successful threesome including advice on dismantling your own preconceptions about sex and love; managing jealousy; developing self-awareness; and communicating openly, honestly, and directly.

A growing cadre of threesome proponents (including psychotherapists, polyamory instructors, relationship gurus, and an assorted lot of self-identified trisexuals) say that threesomes can be improve a couple's relationship by upping the erotic quotient, honing communication skills, deepening intimacy, and defusing overdependency. Couples with a high level of happiness, honesty, communication, and trust often find that threesomes help them reorganize their relationship at a higher level. But this only works when the relationship foundation is already solid. Remember: not all relationships are threesome-proof. If you're feeling insecure about yourself or your relationship, a three-way could leave you feeling used, bitter, or blue. So, before swinging it three-way style, take the time to deactivate the emotional tripwires. Trust me, you'll be glad you did. If you skip this chapter now, refer to it later for damage control.

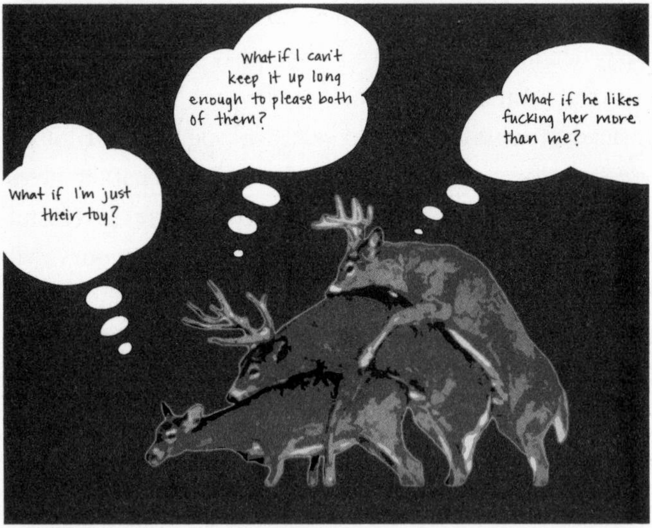
What if I'm just their toy?
What if I can't keep it up long enough to please both of them?
What if he likes fucking her more than me?

The "What Ifs"

STEP 1. FORGET WHAT YOUR MAMA TOLD YOU

I strongly believe that open relationships reduce the hazards that accompany unhealthy codependency. Open relationships challenge us to confront our jealousy and possessiveness. Committing to relationships not mapped out by our parents or society or Hollywood means tearing down the very foundation of status quo and conformity. It means redefining and rebuilding a relationship based on your needs and your values. Loving openly and freely in this day and age is a political act.

—Wendy-O Matik, *Redefining Our Relationships*

Letting go of sexual hang-ups requires some reprogramming. If you're like most of us, your mama didn't teach you that threesomes were wholesome. She probably never sat you down and delineated all the ways that birds and bees can get their groove on—from all-male trios to "closed circle" heteroflexible triads—nor did she champion these sexual expressions as equally valid, legitimate, and beautiful. Most of us have grown up on idyllic images of straight monogamous coupledom. Lonely single finally meets "the one," falls in love, lives happily ever after, and enjoys meaningful monogamy for eternity. This fairy tale seeps into our psyches. In reality, however, romance often takes a different turn; hormones wear off, perfect lovers suddenly reveal flaws, and before long, strangers start looking incredibly sexy. Even those in exquisitely spark-filled, love-oozing committed relationships are likely to meet other captivating hotties. Would it be such a disaster if we all admitted our secret longings?

Desire, it turns out, is a mysterious, mercurial beast that doesn't abide by cultural prescriptions, personal loyalties, or even legal authority. It can spring up unexpectedly during a conversation with someone in a 7-Eleven parking lot at dawn or appear suddenly in a marital bedroom after years of apathy. When desire doesn't conform to our cultural sensibilities, we can choose to repress it or confine ourselves to daydreams. Fortunately, there are alternatives. Thanks to the sexual trailblazers in history, the definitions of acceptable sexual expression have broadened exponentially. Just forty years ago, many states in the United States still banned interracial marriage; thirty-three years ago, the American Psychiatric Association finally declassified homosexuality as a mental illness; and, in July of 2006, Merriam-Webster dictionaries finally included the word *polyamory,* defined as "the state or practice of having more than one open romantic relationship at a time."

But in spite of the smorgasbord of sexual identities to choose from, we all still hold preconceived ideas about what relationships and sex should be like. And when our real sexual desires or relationships don't match up with these images, it's easy to feel ashamed or disappointed. Instead of wondering what's wrong with you, consider what's wrong with dominant ideals and abandon those that don't work. Just because a certain relationship structure is officially sanctioned, doesn't mean it's "natural" or "right." The myths we buy into about "healthy, normal" sex uphold oppressive cultural norms and keep us from living the lives we really want. They're persistent demons, but if you manage to take them down, you may feel empowered to create the life you want. Start by dumping shame and developing a sex-positive attitude.

Society is operating under an illusion right now, meaning what is actually happening in our culture in terms of relationships and sexuality is not being

> accurately reflected in mainstream media. Thousands come to me and Sasha . . . to explore the new paradigms of relating: swinging, tantra, polyamory, bisexuality, etc. They say they must hide their thoughts, desires, and actions from their mates, children, parents, employees, coworkers, society for fear of repercussions. From my perspective as the Dear Abby of the Internet, the revolution is here. While there are many who are celebrating and joyful in their newfound revelation, there are still many times more who suffer because they must hide who they really are behind shame and guilt, which does not accurately reflect the truths of their hearts.
>
> —Janet Lessin, president of the World Polyamory Association

Booting old wives' tales

As you begin your threesome adventures, consider these myths about relationships, gender, and sexuality:

1. Monogamous twosomes are the only healthy, legitimate relationships. While monogamy is the culturally dominant relationship model in America today, it isn't "natural" or "biological," and it isn't the only way to have a relationship. Other societies, past and present, have considered nonmonogamous relationships the norm; in fact, polygamy has been sanctioned by much of the world through extended periods in history, from the biblical Middle East to modern-day Salt Lake City. And with the U.S. divorce rate hovering around 50 percent, it's clear that monogamy isn't panning out perfectly for everyone.

In 2005, Victor de Buijn, his wife Biance, and their lover, Mirjam Geven, were married in a three-way union in the Netherlands.

In the United States, monogamy has long been the default setting for long-term love. When feelings bubble up outside of the marital nest, conventional wisdom tells us we have three choices: extinguish these extracurricular longings, end the existing relationship, or get some booty on the sly (and feel like a sleazy creep). Maybe we can have our cake and eat it, too.

Recently, a growing number of Americans have started reinventing romance by exploring alternative relationship paradigms that promise to be more exiting and fulfilling than the restrictive marriages our parents suffered. Lovers in the new millennium are finding ways to tweak monogamy—from "don't ask, don't tell" policies for extramarital affairs to threesomes (with both partners present) to kiss-and-tell licenses (which permit partners to independently smooch strangers as long as they report home about it). Their motto: Honesty. While American society has long tolerated married men getting some on the sly (with a boys-will-be-boys wink), slutting around is finally becoming an honest, fair, and viable option for both sexes.

Experimenting with new relationship models doesn't mean you've got to trade in your Armani suit for a floral muumuu or move to a nudist commune in Kauai. There's a new breed of hipsters ripping at the seams of monogamy. They're not excessively earnest hippie free-lovers or old-school swingers or social misfits, they're, well . . . cool. Many of these folks don't label themselves as polyamorous or swingers, often preferring the term *modern*. They've updated monogamy to the twenty-first century and tweaked it to fit their own needs and desires. These trendsetters are cropping up in cities all over the nation, and they're leading us to an advanced civilization of romance, gleaming with possibility. Many love revolutionaries have custom designed their own relationship paradigms so brilliantly that knee-jerk monogamists will scratch their heads and wonder how they ever got duped into being so square, so socially programmed, and so old-fashioned. Ball-and-chain style love may be on the way out.

And contrary to the stereotype that couples interested in extramarital booty are sex starved or plain bored, most "modern couples" who swing it three-way style have extremely loving, happy, healthy, and intimate relationships. They've often been together for eons, they're secure in their relationship, and they want each other to experience magic with other fabulous people in the world. Now, that's love.

> Psychological studies show no difference in marital stability between "polyamorous" and monogamous couples; and couples with "open marriages" were found normal in terms of marital satisfaction and self-esteem.[2] In fact, studies show that couples in "open relationships" tend to gain more experience communicating openly and report more satisfaction with their relationships.

Sex and love can take an infinite range of forms—from lesbian trios to straight men who occasionally give other men blowjobs while their wives watch. And these relationships are every bit as valid, good, and healthy as the traditionally accepted monogamous heterosexual couple. So, instead of forcing relationships into predetermined cultural models, consider the infinite possibilities for more love, deeper intimacy, and hotter nooky. And threesomes are an ideal way to start reinventing monogamy.

> Pretending the world is monogamous when it's not is just foolish. If we look at relationships realistically and start asking why we do what we do, we can start thinking of real solutions. That gives me hope for the world. It's better than thinking everyone is an asshole when they cheat. Why can't we all realize that it's healthy to be attracted to other people, instead of trying to ignore it? Honestly, monogamous relationships get kind of boring and threesomes can be an exciting, safe way to enjoy new sexual partners.
>
> —Rachel, 35

Radical Lovers in History

In the 1830s, John Noyes, Yale Divinity School student and theological rebel, declared marriage a "selfish institution in which men exerted rights of ownership over women." Founded on Noyes's theories, the Oneida Community in New York (1848–1879) espoused "complex marriage," whereby all members of the community were married.

Sheep Do It

Male bighorn sheep participate in group sex, where three to ten individuals "cluster together in a circle, rubbing, nuzzling, licking, horning, and mounting each other," according to Bruce Bagemihl in *Biological Diversity,* 1999.

2. If you're really in love, you won't even think about fucking someone else. Get real. Even if your boyfriend is head over heels for you, his cock hasn't lost its nerve endings. Strip the culturally imposed nonsense from the equation and here's what you get: humans like sex and they like variety. There's no monogamy gene (in men or women) and expecting one person to fulfill all of your sexual and emotional needs just isn't realistic. There are plenty of reasons to want to get it on with someone new, even if you're in a phenomenal, committed relationship. Maybe you've been dreaming about getting tied to the bedpost, but your boyfriend doesn't do bondage. Or maybe you occasionally like pussy and your boyfriend doesn't have one. Dump the myth that these smutty cravings mean your honey doesn't love you or that you don't love her, and you're in business.

3. Possessiveness and jealousy are inevitable. Jealousy is an emotion just like any other and it doesn't have to be the tragic mindfuck that most of us seem to think it is.

There's a common assumption that jealousy and love are inextricably intertwined. "If you loved me, you'd be jealous." It's possible to love someone without wanting to own them or control them. Love that isn't possessive feels delicious. Seasoned tri-adventurers say they often feel immense joy at seeing their lovers receive sexual pleasure or love from someone else, without jealousy or fear of loss. In fact, the experience is so common among threesome veterans that they've coined a term for it. *Compersion:* a happy feeling derived from seeing your lover receive affection from someone else.

> Reexamine concepts such as betrayal, cheating, or unfaithfulness, and ask yourself if these still apply to your relationships, how and why. . . . It shouldn't surprise you how filled our heads are with Hollywood's preconceived notions of honor and loyalty. It shouldn't surprise you how indoctrinated we all are in patriarchal concepts of possessiveness. If these institutions are not exposed for the tools of inequality that they are, then we will continue to blindly perpetuate them.
>
> —Wendy-O Matic, *Redefining Our Relationships*

4. Threesomes signal a troubled relationship. There's no reason to assume that threesomes are symptomatic of a crumbling duo. Open relationships can be used as a last-ditch effort to save dying relationships, but just as often this isn't the case. And this myth stunts the possibilities for exploring potentially spectacular alternative relationship choices. The fact is there are so many fascinating people in the world and each one may bring out something new in you. Wanting to get cozy with someone new doesn't mean your existing relationship is a goner.

Plus, relationships that involve nontraditional sexual rules usually require a great deal of communication, honesty, trust, and self-awareness. In fact, couples with solid relationships often find that threesomes actually improve their relationships by challenging them to radically increase their communication skills and honesty. Alternative relationship therapists say that threesomes (and other forms of ethical nonmonogamy) can be a healthy way to alleviate over-dependency, which kills many otherwise good relationships. Many ethically nonmonogamous couples say they don't feel threatened by threesomes because their relationship is so secure and fantastic. (And, many threesome-enthusiast couples have been happily together for decades.) So, don't interpret a threesome as a relationship death knell.

5. Women who have sex outside of monogamous relationships are "sluts." Women are just as horny for new love as men. Of course, there are more sexist cultural restrictions on women's sexual expression—having lots of great sex with a variety of partners warrants being called a slut if you're a woman, lucky if you're a guy. Don't let sexism cramp your style.

> Humans are not a pair-bonding species. Women are promiscuous by nature, desiring more than one mate, and men are even worse.
>
> —Scientist Robert Wright, *Time*

6. I told you so. When something goes awry for threesome explorers, monogamists love to gloat: "I told you so. What did you expect from a three-way?" (Envy can be ugly.) Of course, this is silly reasoning: I would be hoarse if I said, "I told you so, what did you expect from a monogamous twosome?" every time an average couple broke it off. But when sexual adventurers run into rough waters, it's common for monogamists to feel smug. Don't buy into this defeatist attitude. Pat yourself on the back for doing something unconventional, something that requires courage. And if it goes wrong once, that doesn't mean the whole project is doomed. It's common for couples and singles to successfully enjoy three-way flings; and plenty of long-term triad relationships go on happily for decades. Not every threesome experience will work out perfectly, just as not every monogamous relationship will stick forever. Learn from your mistakes and it'll get easier.

7. Having a threesome will make me a bad feminist. A F^2M threesome invariably elicits a big high five from the guys. Others assume that this type of threesome renders women victims of the patriarchy—implying that they've been unwittingly conned into putting on a show for some man's horny two-chick fantasy. This interpretation casts women as passive victims, who don't know what's good for them. While some women participate in threesomes with other women just to please their guy, plenty of women choose threesomes with other women because it gets them wet. Bi-curious and bisexual women, who are hot for the sexy deliciousness of girl sex, get a super-sweet deal with a F^2M threesome. Other F^2M lovers: exhibitionist women who get turned on being watched. There's nothing antifeminist about a woman knowing what she wants in bed and getting it. And, no, F^2M threesomes don't invariably spark competition over the guy. This notion is based on the sexist assumption that women can't cooperate and are inherently prone to catfights over their male love interests. Contrary to gender stereotypes, F^2M threesomes can be an empowering and bonding experience for women. Plus, two women can fuck each other and cum all night long without an erection-restoring break. . . . When you put it that way, the man in the equation may amount to nothing more than a bonus joystick. And, if the sexy threesome turns into a long-term trio relationship, an extra person to share the household chores is likely to catapult career women to the top. Let the bra burning begin.

My friends thought that the second woman in our threesome was "a bonus" for my husband. I guess they assumed I was totally straight and that I cater to my husband's sexual fantasies without getting my own sexual desires met. I'm actually bisexual and I've had plenty of threesomes with two guys, but I prefer bringing in another woman—there's nothing like getting guy loving and soft woman loving at the same time.

—Karin, 29

Feminists for Polygamy

In 1997, lawyer Elizabeth Joseph gave a speech to the National Organization for Women, proclaiming polygamy the "ultimate feminist lifestyle." Joseph said polygamy ensures her kids are well cared for while she's out bringing home the bacon. *Hmm* . . . threesomes a solution for working moms?

Feminists Rock It Three-Way Style, Too

Patricia Ireland, former president of the National Organization for Women (the largest feminist organization in the United States) shared her life with her husband and her female lover. She told the *New York Times* that she hoped the discussion of her personal life helped dispel the myth that most Americans live in traditional families. "There's still this concept of Mom, Dad, Dick, Jane, Spot, Puff. But there are really all kinds of arrangements people make in their lives. . . . Certain people are uncomfortable with it who are otherwise comfortable with feminist issues. But all of us need to be challenged in our thinking. This is how I live my life and I'm not ashamed. Here I am. Here's my whole set of skills. You get the parts of me you like and also the parts that make you uncomfortable."[3]

Ah, for the Life of a Eurasian Oystercatcher

These birds participate in F^2M threesomes. The females share a nest; all mate with each other several times a day; and they preen feathers together. Domestic harmony.

Ask Sally Threesome

Q. Will having a threesome interfere with my religious faith?

A. Even upstanding bible-thumpers swing it three-way style. According to one Web site dedicated to interpreting biblical rules on sexuality (www.Sexinchrist.com), threesomes with two women are perfectly natural. Just more evidence that God really does exist! Christian groups from Texas to Utah say that multiple spouses are exactly what the good Lord intended. Check out "Liberated Christians" at www.libchrist.com. (I mean, if he didn't, why the heck would he have made threesomes so damn hot? That kind of sexy couldn't be the devil's work.) And Christians aren't the only God-fearing folks who see three as God's prerogative. Islam and threesomes go hand-in-hand, too. (Some Islamic sects sanction having two wives, as long as they're both treated equally). Thank you, Mohammed.

Update your core beliefs

Consider this an invitation to let go of outdated core beliefs that no longer serve you. Relationship therapist Kathy Labriola recommends updating these old beliefs with shiny new ones that allow more possibilities in terms of love, sex, and relationships.[4] Try these on for size:

1. My partner loves me so much that (s)he trusts our relationship to expand and be enriched by opening ourselves to even more love from others.
2. My relationship is so solid and trusting that we can bring in a third lover freely. My partner is so satisfied with me and our relationship that bringing in another lover will not threaten our bond.
3. There's an unlimited supply of love in the world. Getting snuggly with more than one person is a choice that can exponentially expand my potential for giving and receiving love, affection, and other sweet treats.

Hmm. Not half bad, eh?

STEP 2. KNOW THYSELF

Clarify what you want and why

There are many reasons to have a threesome. Some tri-curious men and women want to remain "emotionally monogamous" with the added sexual fire of extra hands and tongues. Other couples bring in a third to avoid the "grass is greener" syndrome. Some singles, who have recently gotten out of long-term relationships or marriages, find that threesomes offer them much-needed sexual attention without the pressure of getting involved in a new relationship. Threesomes also offer a safer way to explore bi-curiosity.

Whatever your reasons, it's best to have a clear picture of why you're dreaming of swinging it three-way style. Before hounding your partner to have a threesome or before agreeing to one, clarify your own desires, motives and concerns. Clear your head. Self-awareness is mandatory. Now, dream big: what do you want in terms of sex, love, and intimacy? What's your perfect threesome?

Most importantly, to have a wicked hot threesome, you've got to want it. Check in with yourself. If you're considering a threesome because your boyfriend nagged you or promised you a lifetime supply of peanut brittle, the sex just isn't going to be that good and the fallout is going to be messy. A threesome can be an amazing adventure if you're doing it because you want to—because it's fun, intriguing, sexy, and challenging. If you're doing it for the wrong reasons (i.e., to shut your lover up or to salvage a deteriorating relationship), you'll likely kick yourself later. Being pressured into a threesome could stir enough bitterness and resentment to poison any relationship.

Many people try to live a monogamous lifestyle and find it just does not meet their needs. They find that it's unrealistic to expect any one person to fulfill all their needs for intimacy, companionship, love, and sex, for the rest of their lives. Most people practice "serial monogamy"—having one monogamous relationship after another, swapping out one partner for another when they find each person can't fulfill their needs and dumping each partner when they find themselves dissatisfied. Many people spend their whole lives searching for the perfect mate, only to find themselves dissatisfied time after time. They cannot maintain a monogamous relationship over the long haul, because one partner cheats, loses interest, or one or both partners discover conflicts or incompatible needs. Ethical nonmonogamy can alleviate some of these problems.

—Relationship counselor Kathy Labriola

Shrink's Corner

Consider your own reasons for wanting a threesome. Relationship counselor Kathy Labriola says there are healthy and unhealthy reasons for wanting to explore nonmonogamy.[5] Most people have a mix of both, so don't flog yourself for having some unhealthy motivations, but it's wise to clean up your unhealthy motivations first.

Reasons for wanting to stick to two: For some, monogamy offers the safety to explore deep intimacy with someone. This can be a path of personal growth, which may allow some to work through their issues or childhood pain. But, plenty of people insist on monogamy for unhealthy reasons like a strong need for emotional or financial security. In reality, monogamy doesn't offer an iron-clad security guarantee (witness the 50 percent divorce rate) and fear-based monogamy often translates into a vapid existence.

Reasons for wanting a threesome: Healthy motivations for a three-way include a desire for sexual variety and bisexual lovin'. Other healthy motivations include a desire to overcome fears of abandonment; to conquer jealousy and possessiveness; to learn to express needs clearly; to improve communication skills; or to alleviate overdependency in an existing relationship. However, using a threesome to save a withering relationship or to get high on the buzz of a new relationship isn't healthy. Other unhealthy motivations for a three-way: fear of intimacy and commitment-phobia. Having more than one partner can make commitment-phobes feel safer and allow them to avoid dealing with their own inability to commit. Other unsound threesome motivations: one partner fears the other is dissatisfied and uses a threesome to please him, or one partner wants to leave the relationship but they're too chicken to do it.

Unpack your bags

To get into a three-way without unconsciously dumping your old relationship baggage into the present situation, you need to be willing to unpack those bags from the past. Maybe your ex cheated on you with your best friend and you're still too broken up about it to even consider sharing your current lover with another. Maybe you were raised Catholic and you can't shake the guilt. We've all got some scarring, but if you're too insecure or you've got huge emotional wounds that you've been repressing for thirty years, try to work through those obstacles before having a three-way. Threesomes feel best when you're feeling good about yourself and when you're open to learning from whatever comes up.

Three-ways have a remarkable way of shining spotlights on our rawest emotional trigger-points. That's part of what's potentially so transformative about them. So, enter the terrain with curiosity and a willingness to investigate whatever the experience brings up for you (even the uncomfortable stuff). Threesomes present a unique opportunity to get past basic insecurities and deeply discover that you're truly lovable. So, welcome whatever emotional whirlwinds get activated in you. Be curious about them. Investigate. Be willing to unpack these bags as they surface, rather than just shoving them in the closet.

> You have baggage that you carry with you, even if you are a virtual candidate for sainthood. All of us odd little humans carry our load of hopes, dreams, and wishes, as well as fears and doubts. Developing the ability to ferret them out, to look at them with both objectivity and sympathy, and deal with them is not only recommended, but necessary to being responsibly nonmonogamous.
>
> —Anthony Ravenscroft, *Polyamory: Roadmaps for the Clueless & Hopeful*

Be brave, curious, and compassionate

As you start exploring threesomes, you will, undoubtedly, face some fears. You might find that you're gayer than you thought. Or ancient fears of being unlovable or unattractive will surface. Maybe you'll worry that there won't be enough love for you. It's okay; don't flinch. Instead of rushing back into your comfort zone, challenge yourself to relax into the uncomfortable feelings, experience them, and maybe even enjoy the ride. So, instead of shrieking and crawling back into safety when you hit an emotionally uncomfortable pothole, enter the three-way terrain with a curious attitude and a sense of discovery about what you'll learn about yourself. Going against the mainstream requires an enormous amount of courage. Consider using your threesome adventure to become a warrior—to practice bravery, to learn to communicate clearly and openly, and to navigate unfamiliar territory. Stretching comfort zones requires tolerating some discomfort at the beginning. If you're willing to face whatever comes up for you, you'll grow from the experience.

At any point, your fearful paranoid mind could pull you into the darkest spots inside yourself—the place where you're entirely convinced that you're a chump or the third wheel. "You've been duped! You're likely to get deserted here." That insecure mind may call out. Threesomes offer a bizarrely powerful opportunity to see the mind's fluctuation between twin impulses of fear and love, in action. Once your insecure paranoia settles, you may find your soul venturing down another path—one that swells with big love that isn't possessive or jealous or insecure. In those moments, you may feel entirely lovable, bursting with enough love for everyone on the planet, and open an ability to receiving lots of love. It takes an enormous amount of courage to see that fearful paranoid mind and accept those emotions as just emotions flowing through and allow them to pass through you, without shutting down in fear. Instead, practice allowing yourself to open in uncomfortable, risky ways. Threesomes can stretch our ability to love—use your threesome to practice observing and accepting your own fearful mind, and still allowing yourself to open even when fear makes you feel like closing up. Learning to open to love without trying to freeze it into a rigid form that's identifiable, socially acceptable, and secure takes practice, but you may feel remarkably open and alive. Relish it.

> Confess your hidden faults.
> Approach what you find repulsive.
> Help those you think you cannot help.
> Anything you are attached to, let it go.
> Go to places that scare you.
>
> —Advice from Tibetan Yogini Machik Labdron
> in *The Places That Scare You,* Pema Chodron

Don't put on a show, unless it makes you hot

Threesomes offer ideal exhibitionist opportunities. Having a threesome to put on a two-girl show for your guy can be wicked hot. If strutting your stuff for an audience makes you wet, encore. But check in with yourself. If you're dyking out just to satisfy someone else's fantasy, consider getting your own sexual fantasies fulfilled.

Get clear

Meditation is one way to get a clear head. There are hundreds of styles; the ones I like best use the physical body to develop self-awareness. Observing physical sensations can help you release old patterns, move through uncomfortable emotions, and observe yourself. Focusing on body and breath is one way to go beneath the words into a nonverbal experience of emotions. Instead of using meditation to bliss out to avoid pain, use it to become more aware of your own mind and emotional terrain. Meditation teaches us to stay open to whatever arises (whether pleasant or unpleasant), experience it, accept it, and let it go. To learn more, take a class in mindfulness, insight meditation, or vipassana. Meditation centers around the country offer courses, some free or low-cost (www.dhamma.org, www.dharma.org, www.insightmeditation.org), others with a high price tag (www.spiritrock.org). Body-oriented therapists use similar techniques. Others swear by transcendental meditation (www.tm.org). If meditating isn't your cup of tea, find out what works for you—consider yoga, running, or therapy.

Self-awareness exercises

1. **For a little taste of meditation, start by noticing your breath.** Observe if it's heavy, fast, slow, or shallow. Can you feel it hitting a spot under your nostrils? Don't try to control or change your breath, just observe it. When your thoughts wander, patiently bring your attention back to the breath. When emotional distress arises, try to allow the thoughts or the story line to pass and return to an awareness of your breath. Take a meditation workshop.

2. **Make a list of your threesome fears.** Look in the mirror and say, "I'm good enough, I'm smart enough, and gosh darn it, I deserve a hot three-way."

3. **Review Your Self-Awareness.**

- Do you consider threesomes a legitimate and healthy form of sexual expression?
- Are you aware of your own relationship or sexuality hang-ups that might dampen your three-way bliss?
- Are you clear on your own reasons for wanting a threesome?
- Are you clear on your fears about a threesome? Are you prepared to confront them?
- Are you feeling excited about a threesome adventure?
- Do you feel sexy and secure?

- Do you feel that you've made your own choice about having a threesome or that you've been pressured into it?
- Are you prepared to work through any challenging emotions that come up during the adventure and use them as an opportunity for personal growth?

STEP 3. THE BIG J: NIP JEALOUSY IN THE BUD (OR LET IT GET YOU HOT)

> My girlfriend has learned that jealousy actually enhances her own plumbing, so she's learned to enjoy her own jealousy. It won't go away, even after ten years of doing threesomes. There are going to be times when you're triggered to be jealous. In that moment you can go into fear and get stuck in your own matrix of insecurity or you can pull your panties down and check your pussy and notice that it's wet. . . . And, you have to ask yourself, can you enjoy that wetness and jump in? That will make or break a threesome.
>
> —Stephane Hemon, seduction guru

Jealousy's a bitch. And it's a legitimate concern for novice threesome explorers and seasoned vets alike. The good news: jealousy is an emotion that can be unlearned and even if it can't be entirely eradicated, you'll be much stronger and cooler if you learn to handle it. Jealousy can feel overwhelmingly gut-wrenching, but with practice and a few tools, you can learn to manage it with grace. If you're exploring threesomes, jealousy could crop up. Accept that this might be part of the journey and commit to learning from it. If you're prepared to confront any emotions that get stirred up and to communicate about them directly, jealousy can be an opportunity for personal growth and greater intimacy with your primary partner. Learning to manage jealousy can lead you to a sweet spot inside yourself, where you feel so confident that you no longer seek validation from anyone else. And that's a beautiful thing.

If you could untie your wings
And free your soul of jealousy,

You and everyone around you
Would fly up like doves.

—Jalal ad-Din Rumi,
Persian poet and mystic

I really have my jealousy under control. I still get jealous, but if I get jealous, it involves a crunch

> feeling in my heart and gut for about five seconds, then it's gone. As soon as I start feeling upset about it, I remind myself that what I have with this person stands on its own. I always think of a mother who loves one child, then gives birth to a second child. That doesn't require her to love her first child any less. Once you establish a bond with someone, it's not going to go away or diminish, because you both find someone else. This is what I tell people who are shocked or even offended when I talk about polyamory. A human being is capable of loving more than one person at a time.
>
> —Daniel, 29

Strategies for managing jealousy

1. Assess the situation. Check your relationship with your boyfriend: is it solid and committed? Evaluate the third: do you feel he/she has sinister motives? Does the third respect your relationship with your partner? If there isn't a legitimate threat, it can be rewarding to work through any jealousy that arises.

2. Acknowledge it. When you feel jealous, recognize it in yourself. Jealousy can be overpowering, so it's helpful to commit not to act on it, even if you feel the overwhelming urge to bust someone's jaw. Fooling yourself into thinking you're not jealous when you are can lead you to "act out" indirectly and that's damned unhelpful. While our normal impulse might be to avoid or repress painful emotions, the best way to handle jealousy is to acknowledge it and allow yourself to feel it. It will hurt. Accept it. Don't down a fifth of Jack to avoid feeling it. Will you feel shitty? Probably. Will it kill you? Probably not. And you may feel like a superhero if you learn to handle challenging emotions like jealousy.

3. Observe it physically. One technique for confronting jealousy is to use your body. Most emotions can be felt as physical sensations. When I get jealous, I feel tension in my jaw, queasiness in my stomach, heat in my chest, and a range of other unpleasant sensations. Paying attention to physical sensations (and breath) can make it easier to move through difficult feelings. During this exercise, don't get caught up in the story line about why you're feeling jealous, just keep bringing your attention back to your body. Observe the physical sensations attached to jealousy, feel it, experience the pain of it, and accept it. It's challenging to be in the space we usually want to avoid—the uncomfortable, painful spot. And, learning to move toward our emotional distress can be transformative; if we allow the experience to soften us, rather than make us bitter. Watch it and let it flow, knowing that it'll pass.

> When we touch the center of sorrow, when we sit with discomfort without trying to fix it, when we stay present to the pain of disapproval or betray and let it soften us, these are the times that we connect with [our compassionate selves]. Tapping into that shaky and tender place has a transformative effect.
>
> —Pema Chodron, *The Places That Scare You*

4. Spend time with your rival. Another strategy for defusing jealousy is to spend time with the person inspiring your jealous feelings. Veteran three-way lovers find that getting to know the threatening person tends to melt jealousy. One twenty-five-year-old bisexual woman, who's been having threesomes for years, summed it up: "I find that interacting more with the new person helps me feel less jealous. Even if it's a superficial connection, when I get to know the person, I feel better. Getting to know the person helps me realize that she has flaws and she's not this scary perfect woman that I've created in my mind."

5. Think about it. After you've calmed down, consider why jealousy surfaced. Try to figure out where it's coming from and what it can teach you about yourself or your relationship. Jealousy can spring up because you're feeling insecure about yourself, or because you're not getting your needs met in your relationship, or because you want to be the best at everything so the mere possibility that someone else might give a better blowjob than you makes your blood boil. Jealousy can also surface when old emotional scars from past relationships are triggered. Let jealousy guide you into yourself to find pain that needs healing.

> Let jealousy be your teacher. Jealousy can lead you to the very places where you need healing. It can be your guide into your own dark side and show you the way to total self-realization. Jealousy can teach you how to live in peace with yourself and with the whole world if you let it.
>
> —Dr. Deborah Anapol, *Polyamory: The New Love Without Limits*

If the mere thought of having a threesome and watching your lover kiss someone else gives you the shakes, consider what bugs you about it. There's usually some concoction of fear, anger, or powerlessness hiding under jealousy. Often jealousy stems from fear of loss or abandonment. Relationship therapist Kathy Labriola advises trying to unmask jealousy:

> I try to help them identify the primary emotion behind the jealousy. Is it fear? Sadness? Anger? For most people, behind jealousy, there's an emotion . . . and usually it's fear of loss. There's usually an unmet need behind that jealousy and I try to help them figure out how they can get that need met to feel happy and safe in a relationship.

Are you feeling sex-deprived by your partner and scared that an extra person might mean even less booty for you? Maybe you're worried that your lover will dump you for someone with better moves and a tighter ass. If that's a legitimate threat, then your relationship needs some work; if it's not a legitimate threat, consider doing some work on your own. Jealousy can be a perfect invitation to confront your insecurities head-on and to realize just how lovable, attractive, and beautiful you are. That's a tall order, but it's possible.

If you're getting what you need in your relationship, you'll be less likely to feel jealous during a threesome—even when your partner has sex with another person (you might even find yourself feeling really happy about it). If you're getting enough hot sex from your partner, it's less likely to sting when it happens with someone else. Consider friendships: you probably don't feel jealous when your best friend plays foosball with another friend, unless you've been feeling neglected. Romantic relationships work similarly. So, if jealousy surfaces, let it raise questions for you about whether you're getting your needs met in your relationship. When jealousy stems from feelings of deprivation in a relationship, it's best to iron that out before bringing in another partner so that both partners feel there's enough love to go around.

6. Own it. It's easy to slip into blaming someone else when you feel jealous. By owning jealous feelings, you empower yourself to take control of your situation and make changes where changes are due. If you feel jealous, own it. Remember, it's your job to get what you need in your relationships, so take responsibility. If you're upset that your lover doesn't tickle your pearl anymore, it's up to you to ask.

> Jealousy makes the prick grow harder and the cunt wetter.
>
> —Erica Jong, *How to Save Your Life*

7. Use jealousy to adjust your limits. Once you figure out where your jealousy is coming from, negotiate an agreement that would make you feel safer in your relationship so that you can comfortably explore a threesome. Once you know what scares you, you can face it, express it, and negotiate an agreement that makes you feel safer about potentially jealousy-inducing situations. In other words, if imagining a threesome makes you jealous because you're scared you'll lose your lover, ask yourself how you could feel safer about that prospect. Would it help if your lover verbally agreed to sever all ties with a third if you made the request? Would it help if your lover committed to not having any physical contact with the third when you aren't around (be specific: does this mean you don't want them spooning while you're taking a bathroom break, or does it mean you don't want them fucking when you're out of town)?

Instead of diving into a situation that you know will spark a jealousy whirlwind in yourself, try gradually increasing your limits as you become more comfortable. Step by step, by acknowledging your own jealousy and communicating about it directly, you'll be empowered to strip the motor out of it.

8. Say it. Once you know what's going on inside yourself, communicate honestly and directly. If you feel jealous, tell your partner. That might be embarrassing, but do it anyway. If you pretend you're not jealous when you are, your partner can't help you feel more secure and you can't ask for what you need. Withholding when you feel jealous is a sure way to make the situation worse. If you share it with your lover, you'll have an easier time negotiating a threesome that feels safe for both of you. Then tell your lover what you need from him. A seasoned threesome explorer said, "When jealousy comes up for me, I ask my husband to make me feel important, like I'm wanted, like I'm interesting as well as this sparkling new person. You have to say what you need in order to get what you need." One novice threesome explorer explained that telling her partner about her jealousy right away, solved the problem:

> My boyfriend and I were at a bar hitting on this friend we were interested in having a threesome with. I suddenly realized that I felt jealous because he seemed to be giving her too much attention. In high-school drama mode, I probably would have started acting bitchy or tried to make them both jealous by leaving with another guy. Instead, I just whispered in his ear: "Pay a little more attention to me, sweetness."And it felt fantastic. He was so happy that I told him and was more than happy to show me his affection—he was just trying to make

> the new person feel included and adored. Just after I whispered that to him, she turned around and planted a juicy kiss on my lips.
>
> —Elan, 34

Final words on jealousy

Jealousy can be an amazing learning tool. It can guide you to insecurities in yourself that need to be handled and snags in your relationships that need to be addressed. Be grateful that it appeared and use it wisely. If you listen to it and confront it, you'll reap big rewards. Beyond discovering how lovable and beautiful you are, you might learn to love bigger without needing to control or own someone. Those who've gotten jealousy management down say they often feel deep happiness when their lover gets an incredible hummer from someone else or experiences emotional intimacy with another lover. There's certainly enough love to go around, so it's worth peeling away our own insecurities to step into the love stream with open arms.

Jealousy Don'ts

Don't pretend you're not jealous if you are.

Don't get drunk or high to numb the pain.

Don't act on it.

Don't blame someone else.

Don't take it as a license to be abusive.

Jealousy Dos

Acknowledge it.

Welcome it as an opportunity to understand yourself better.

Observe it.

Accept that it's painful.

Try to figure out why you're feeling it.

Tell your partner about it.

Explain what you need from your partner without blaming.

Know it will pass.

Be forgiving.

Jealousy Management Exercises

Spend ten minutes on this pre-threesome jealousy prevention exercise. Write down your thoughts on the following topics and share them with each other.

1. Be self-aware. Think about jealousy on your own. Imagine a threesome scenario that might generate jealousy. Be specific.

2. Make a jealousy pact. Commit to tell each other when you feel jealous and to ask for reassurance when you need it. Agree that if one partner feels jealous, the other will listen, sympathize, and validate (rather than, scream or insist on "fixing it").

3. Discuss how to make a threesome feel safest for both of you.

4. Set comfortable limits and stick to them (see page 167).

5. Develop codes to communicate with each other during your threesome (see page 173). That way, if either of you start feeling jealous, you'll be able to communicate directly and immediately about it and change the situation.

6. Review the section on choosing the right third. Discuss people who you'd both feel least jealous inviting into bed (see chapter 3).

STEP 4. COMMUNICATE, COMMUNICATE, COMMUNICATE

Sure, you'd happily donate a kidney to have a threesome, but if you're in a relationship and your partner doesn't feel good about, it's not going to be a positive experience. There's a risk of awkward sex and relationship-crushing drama, unless you're both totally onboard. The best way to do this is to figure out your own needs, desires, and concerns; express yourself clearly and honestly to your partner; encourage your partner to fully express herself;

then negotiate a solution that works for both of you. You're going to need to learn to talk to each other honestly (and productively) about difficult and sensitive topics. Here's some essential advice for honing your communication skills so you can negotiate a threesome that works for both of you. . . .

> My husband and I have been together for seven years and we've had lots of threesomes. What allows us to do this? Good communication, knowing where our boundaries are, and confidence in our connection. I know my husband loves me. I feel that bond and I know I'm irreplaceable. After seven years, I can say that. We treat each other well and we recognize the third person as a playmate. We're always honest with the third person about our expectations and we take care of them too, so that makes them positive experiences.
>
> —Christine, 33

> Threesomes would be as much a study of communication styles as sexual gymnastics.
>
> —Arno Karlen, threesome scholar

A house built on a weak foundation . . .

If you're in a committed relationship, make sure your house is in order first. All change generates some stress in relationships, so going from two to three will create some hiccups. Make sure your relationship is happy, stable, and strong enough to tolerate some stress. "In many heterosexual relationships, the woman feels like she's not getting enough love, attention, affection, romance, intimacy, acknowledgment, and recognition of who she is. So, when the man says he wants to have another partner, if the woman already feels deprived in the relationship, she might worry that she'll get even less if another woman is involved," says relationship counselor, Kathy Labriola. In this situation, alternative relationship counselors recommend fixing the primary relationship first. When both partners feel a sense of abundance of love and attention, they're more likely to feel good sharing their lover. So, if something's broken in your relationship, fix it before inviting a third into the bedroom. Seduction guru Stephane Hemon, who has threesomes with his girlfriend, advises couples to fix their relationships first:

> It's all about trust and a lot of couples don't have that trust. They're trying to enhance their relationship by bringing in a third girl, rather than already having a solid foundation. They're trying to fill a void in their relationship with another girl. Like, "Oh, we're bored, let's try to make this exciting." If you're bored in your relationship, you better figure

out why and fix that, because shit can get complicated with a third.

Tales from the Dark Side: Threesomes that Flopped

Threesomes without adequate communication, trust and honesty can flop. Prepare properly.

I got into it with my girlfriend and some guy she met. It started off well; we both played with her tits and fingered her ass. Then when the pants came off, I discovered that the other guy was a total fucking beast in the pants. He upstaged me totally. She started going wild on his cock and I struggled to keep hard by jacking off and massaging her ass, while she sucked him off. After that, she started fucking his brains out and I was totally left out. I was a fucking ghost. I put my pants on and left before they finished. She was my girlfriend for a year and I haven't talked to her since.

—Peter, 23

I had a threesome with my boyfriend and a woman. I had to go to the bathroom, so I left. When I came back, they were going at it on my bed. I felt left out and so mad. I had a fit.

—Valerie, 32

> I had a threesome once with a lesbian couple. It was terrible. I was fucking the femme, while the butch was going down on her. When she started coming (and she was screaming and shit), the butch got pissed and said she couldn't take it anymore and left the room. I felt bad so I stopped. I guess the femme was just checking out the lesbian scene and she was still into men, so the three-way brought up trouble between them.
>
> —Brad, 26

Know what you need

Finding out that your girlfriend wants to bring in another guy can be surprising and it may bring up some insecurities. Consider what you need to feel safe, loved, and happy in a relationship. Whether you need to know that you're the priority over any third party or that your lover won't ditch you for the third, figure out what would make you feel safest in a threesome scenario. Once you know what you need, you can talk to your partner about how to get those needs met.

Don't manipulate

In many couples, one partner is more enthusiastic about a threesome than the other. Resist the temptation to hound your partner. Instead of using pressure tactics or indirectly trying to manipulate your partner, directly state your desires and needs. If you both honestly put your concerns and desires on the table, you can work toward a solution that makes you both feel excited and safe. When both people feel they've participated fully in the decision-making process, it's easier for both to take responsibility and to avoid the blame game if things go awry. What doesn't work: a guy decides he wants a threesome, so his girlfriend goes along with it; the guy decides his girlfriend should kiss women, so she goes along with it; the guy also decides no men should be considered as potential threesome candidates, so she goes along with it. Decision making needs to be shared between equal powers for threesomes to work fabulously for everyone.

One strategy for fair decision making is to imagine your own ideal threesome scenario and your "bottom line" (a least favorite scenario that would still make you happy). Example: Tom's ideal scenario is a long-term threesome sex arrangement with his current partner and his ex-girlfriend. Tom's bottom line (that would still fulfill his threesome fantasy): hearing his current girlfriend talk dirty to him about threesome fantasies while the two of them fuck. His girlfriend's ideal scenario: never having a threesome and never discussing it again. Her bottom line: introducing threesome stories as part of their dirty-talk repertoire as long he promises not to pester her about having a real-life threesome. By sharing dream scenarios and bottom lines, couples often find a sweet middle ground without railroading one partner into agreement.

Innovative Ways to Persuade Your Girlfriend . . .

In May 2006, a man made a bet with his girlfriend: if he could get 2 million hits on his Web site, she would participate in a threesome with another woman. Within two months, after his ménage plea made its way through e-mail forward chains, his site registered more than 13 million hits. Let's hope she paid up.

The truth will set you free

If you want to fulfill your sexual desires and develop lasting relationships, tell each other the truth. This sounds basic, but most of us don't do it. We tell little white lies to protect our loved ones or half-truths to make ourselves look better or we withhold details that might hurt someone. Truth is actually a radical step for most romantic relationships. And telling the truth requires taking emotional risks.

Satisfying relationships are built on trust, which requires an abnormal amount of honesty. Tell each other the truth even if it's inconvenient, even if you're afraid your lover will leave you, even if your lover will be hurt or angry, even if it means telling your lover that you fucked his best friend and it was the best sex you've ever had. Don't hide other friendships, crushes, or attractions. Telling the truth also means admitting your attractions to other people, and other things you might be ashamed of. Basically, it means being honest about the ugly stuff, the stuff that you think might render you unlovable. Resist the urge to tell your lover what you think they want to hear. Pretending you feel great about a situation when you don't, simply can't lead to a fulfilling relationship or a happy threesome encounter. Even seemingly innocuous white lies are debilitating—they block intimacy and slowly eat away at relationships. So bite the bullet. If your relationship can't weather honesty, it can't weather a threesome.

> The first time I kissed a woman, I was at a party. I immediately called my husband from the bathroom to tell him how it went. That level of honesty is perfect for us, plus it was a big turn-on.
>
> —Tina, 26

The first time my husband and I had a threesome with a guy, it was clear that my husband didn't have his shit worked out. He started acting standoffish and said he was going to sleep and we should do "whatever we wanted." I realized that he was going to act pouty the next day, so I told the other guy to stop. When I asked my husband about it the next day, he said he felt used and that the other guy was just trying to get to me. I talked to the other guy and he told me that he found my husband sexy, too, and just wasn't sure how he felt about being touched by a guy. After clearing that up, we've all had some really amazing threesomes together. You can't just roll with stuff. You need to talk about these things.

—Monica, 29

With clear communication, all of your relationships will change, not only with your partner, but with everyone else. You won't need to make assumptions because everything becomes so clear. This is what I want; this is what you want. If we communicate in this way, our world becomes impeccable.

—Don Miguel Ruiz,

The Four Agreements: A Toltec Wisdom Book

Tell Each Other What You're Thinking

Give each other the full set of data so you can each make informed decisions. Here's a sample conversation:

> JUDY: How do you feel about having a three-way with our neighbor, Jack?
>
> TOM: Okay, he's pretty cute. That sounds fine.

Or Tom could say what he's actually thinking . . .

> TOM: Yeah, I find Jack attractive, too, and the threesome sex would probably be a blast, but I feel like he has a crush on you, and he might try to snag you for himself. If he does, will you tell him to get lost? (Now, that's more like it.)

One of my clients was cheating on her husband and couldn't take lying to him anymore. Even though she was terrified, she decided to tell her husband, whom she still loved and had no interest in leaving. She just happened to fall in love with another man as well. We talked a lot about how to tell her husband. She was certain he wouldn't understand because he's very traditional and he'd be hurt. But, when she told him, her husband accepted her new male lover and now they're a triad! It's astonishing. She handled the situation very well after royally screwing it up. Obviously, it doesn't always work this way.

—Bob McGarey, alternative relationship coach
and author of *The Poly Communication Survival Kit*

Ask for what you want

Avoid passive-aggressive behavior by expressing your needs directly and clearly, without expecting your lover to read your mind. It's your responsibility to figure out what you want and to express it honestly and directly. If you spend your energy imagining what your partner wants, instead of deciding what you want, you won't be fulfilled. Start with yourself. And don't assume that your partner will psychically divine your wishes. Expecting your partner to "just know" leads to trouble. Just because you ask, doesn't mean you'll get what you want, but it's critical to learn to ask for what you want directly and clearly. You're much less likely to get what you want if you don't ask for it.

Warning: Getting into a threesome without paying attention to your own desires, needs, and limits, can lead to bitterness and resentment for not getting as much as the other two did out of the three-way. It's your job to get your own needs met, so figure out what they are and go for it.

Know how to say no

To get the most out of a three-way, you need to know when to say no. There are two situations when you should say no: when you don't want to do something and when you're unsure about whether you want to do something. Changing a no to a yes is easy, but you can't take back something you've already done. If you don't feel comfortable saying no, you might agree to something you'll resent later. Become an expert at saying no; that way, when you say yes, you really mean it. Saying no can be a real bitch if you haven't practiced it and it's a critical skill, especially when it comes to navigating new sexual and relationship territory. One way to say no, without worrying about rejecting someone, is to say "not now." Saying no is also a great way to develop trust. When you trust your lovers to tell you the truth about what they do and don't want, it's much easier to feel free asking. To practice: next time you're in a sexual situation, say "not now" or no at some point, just to get comfortable enforcing your boundaries. No need for excuses or apologies, just say no.

Talk about sex

Even long-term couples may not be eager to talk about sex honestly. Couples often feel like they can't be completely honest about their secret desires, especially when they're attracted to others. There's no place for withholds in threesomes—tell your partner the truth about your turn-ons. Whatever it is, tell your lover. But just because you've expressed it doesn't mean your partner will agree to fulfill your fantasy.

Build trust

Trust is an essential threesome building block. And, it doesn't just happen; it's an ongoing process, facilitated by honest communication. If you're in a relationship, you need to trust your partner not to drop you for the next hottie that comes along. Couples who bring in thirds successfully rant and rave about their high level of trust with each other. One thirty-year-old man who's had several threesomes with his long-term girlfriend said that trust makes it possible, "The trust has to be so strong. Imagine trusting your boyfriend so much that when you know he's out on a date with another woman who is physically even more attractive than you, and knowing that he'll drop her like a hot rock if she tries to come between you two." If trust isn't properly established between a couple, a threesome could chip away at the relationship or catalyze a breakup. One way to build trust is to communicate honestly, directly, and clearly—even with ugly insecurities that you'd rather hide in a dusty corner of your mind and not share with anyone. Another way to build trust is to develop boundaries and stick to them.

Create boundaries in advance

If you're not sure how you feel about your boyfriend playing ass-monkey with your neighbor, give him the heads-up in advance. Obviously, you can't predict how you're going to feel in the moment, but it's smart to spend some time clearly defining your boundaries *before* winding up in the sack with a third. Get your permission slip signed before the field trip. If you set limits and communicate them clearly to each other in advance, you're less likely to feel bitter the morning after. Know how far you're both willing to go with a third before you start getting sweaty together. Ask each other: Is there anything you can conceive of that would upset you? Ask yourself: Would it upset me if my partner kissed the third? Would I get upset if we had a threesome and my partner continued schtooping the third, while I went to the loo? Are some activities okay under certain circumstances, but not others? Be specific. Make your limits crystal clear ahead of time. One thirty-eight-year-old man who's been married for fifteen years and regularly enjoys threesomes with his wife explained their success:

> Our relationship is the most important thing in the world. End of story. You've got to really communicate way in advance because in the heat of the moment, you might do something because it's hot and get upset later. We don't assume anything. I

> would have assumed it was okay for me to kiss another woman, but for my wife, it wasn't. It's okay for me to go down on another woman, but not kiss her. So that's a set boundary that we have.

Once you're clear on your own limits, make agreements with your partner before your first threesome. Setting limits and sticking to them will build trust in your relationship. You don't need to dive in with both feet the first time. Take baby steps. The best first-threesome scenario is one that leaves everyone feeling good and eager to try again. When both of you uphold your agreements, your limits will change over time as your trust builds. For example, many couples had very strict limits for their first threesomes, and when those went well, they felt comfortable changing them. (Maybe initially one partner wasn't allowed to kiss the third person, but after several successful threesomes, they renegotiated and kissing is allowed.)

> The first time I had a threesome with my boyfriend and another woman, we agreed in advance that he wasn't going to have intercourse with her. I just wasn't sure I'd be okay with that, so we decided to keep that boundary. After several awesome threesomes, I decided I felt comfortable with my boyfriend having

sex with her. Now, I can't believe how much I get off on watching him make love to other women—that's what makes threesomes so appealing to me.

—Andrea, 29

Know that it's okay to set different boundaries. It's likely that each of you will feel comfortable with different actions—so, it's cool to set different limits. For example: Mary gets turned on watching Tom penetrate other women (so, she's given him the green light on that), but she's not okay with him kissing other women. Tom is uncomfortable with Mary being penetrated by other men, but he's okay with her blowing other men. So, they have different limits and that's just dandy. What's important is that they've each clearly expressed their own limits.

My girlfriend and I met this woman at a party. She was witty, sexy, and funny . . . and she was hitting on both of us. After flirting for a while, the three of us got naked. The experience started out hot, but it ended with hurt feelings, confusion, and upset all around. Basically, our first threesome sucked. My girlfriend and I had talked about threesomes, but we didn't know how to proceed in a real-life three-way.

> It wasn't until we talked about what we each wanted honestly and established clear limits, that we started having amazing threesome experiences.
>
> —Matt, 32

When people don't make clear agreements ahead of time, often someone gets blamed and hurt feelings explode afterward. Sometimes the only way to find out what your limits are, is to cross them and that can be painful. You might think it's okay for your lover to kiss someone else, but find yourself feeling hurt and betrayed. That doesn't mean the whole encounter was a bust. It might mean that you thought you were ready for something that you're not ready for and your limits need to be revised.

> One of our limits is to only have sex with someone else when we're together. We had a threesome with a lesbian, then I had a date with her afterwards. That worried my boyfriend. I was a little too excited about the other woman, so we decided that encroached on our

> relationship boundaries and that we would limit our sexual adventures with others to when we're together.
>
> —Susanna, 29

> I had been fantasizing about seeing my wife make out with another woman for ages, but the first time I saw my wife making the expressions she only made with me with someone else, I was a bit shocked. We left early that night; I had to process it. The next day, I was fine, and we've had dozens of hot threesomes since then, but there are occasional moments like that.
>
> —Ken, 35

There are various ways to create limits that make both parties feel safest about including a third. Sometimes, it helps to get a commitment about how much time will be spent with the new lover or to promise only to use condoms with the third party or to agree to end contact with the third person if the relationship with the third person becomes to intense. It can help to ask your partner to agree that all sexual contact will happen only when both partners are present. Consider what you need to feel secure with your partner and ask for it.

A Sample Agreement That Worked for One Couple

1. Vampire rule. When you're out scamming on potential three-way playmates solo, be back by dawn.

2. All potential three-way playmates must be interested in both members of the couple. Up to three solo dates are allowed to warm them up.

3. Bisexual-men-only rule. (The male member of the couple is bisexual and the woman isn't.)

4. Veto rule. Either member of the couple can rule out potential home wreckers, no questions asked.

5. Only have sex with another person when both members of the couple are present.

6. Safer sex rule. Use condoms during sex with another person.

The basic operating principle: they're a team and that comes before anything.

Critical Pre-Threesome Prep

Create a detailed sex checklist of all the activities that are okay and not okay with a third party. If you're unsure about something, consider it a no. Talk about it. Agree to uphold certain boundaries. Note: you don't need to have logical explanations for why certain activities bother you, while others don't. It's enough to know that certain activities would upset the other person. Agree to respect these limits. Know that your boundaries can and will change over time.

Take responsibility for your choices

If you've made clear agreements ahead of time and you both stick to those limits, then if there's a post-threesome upset, the person feeling upset will be more likely to take responsibility for their emotions instead of blaming anyone. Once you make a decision, own it. If you clearly laid out your limits with your partner and he observes them, but you still end up feeling betrayed or hurt, then it's your responsibility to handle your emotions. Your lover might talk with you about your emotions, but he doesn't need to feel responsible for your bad feelings. And don't blame your lover. After all, if you didn't know in advance that seeing your boyfriend lick another woman's foot would upset you, how could he know? One thirty-five-year-old man felt crummy when his girlfriend ate pussy: "I wasn't expecting to feel jealous when my girlfriend went down on another woman. In fact, I told my girlfriend ahead of time that it was okay. Then when it actually happened, I felt like shit. We talked about it and I realized I was only okay with her kissing other women." Know that it's okay to change your boundaries, if something unexpected ruffles your feathers.

Develop code words in advance

So, you diligently completed your threesome prep activities and you're hitting it with a third you picked up at Starbucks. What if you change your mind? What if you feel left out? Don't expect your significant other to read your mind. If you're feeling left out, don't pout or play passive-aggressive. Develop codes so you can express yourselves clearly during the experience. Code words are essential for couples trying a threesome for the first time. Before things get too hot, make sure to use code words to check in with each other. And keep checking in with each other. This allows you to communicate clearly without assuming the other person is okay with whatever is going on. For example, you could establish *red* as the code word to use if you feel upset and need to stop, *yellow* for "proceed with caution," and *green* for "yeah, baby." Another option: an elbow pinch means "slow down," an armpit pinch means "get me out of here," and a kiss on the palm means "I'm into it." The S/M community considers "safe words" a prerequisite for S/M play. They work like a charm for threesomes, too.

Develop Code Words for the Following

Are you okay with what's going down right now?

I'm freaking out, get me out of here. (If you get this: don't ask questions, just leave ASAP).

I'm a little uncomfortable, slow down with the third.

I'm digging it. Let's keep going.

Ask, listen, and create a solution

Learning to express yourself clearly and to listen to your lover is critical to a happy relationship and a happy threesome. Agree to share 50/50 responsibility for a solution and be willing to be wrong. Once you've expressed your own needs, ask what your partner wants. When both partners feel they have full expressed themselves, it's easier to make collaborative decisions that satisfy both parties, instead of one person giving in to satisfy the other. Bring your partner into the decision-making process by asking open-ended questions (instead of yes or no questions), such as: What does your threesome fantasy look like? What are your concerns? Don't make assumptions about what the other person needs or wants, just ask and keep asking until you understand clearly.

Many of us haven't honed our listening skills. Try this: instead of immediately responding to your partner, try summarizing what's been said and asking if you understand correctly. Repeat this process until your partner feels he has fully expressed himself. Take turns. This parroting technique facilitates better listening skills. Use it, it works.

Request and offer reassurance

If you're opening your relationship to a third, you need to be able to ask for reassurance when you need it. Don't let insecurities boil. There's no shame in asking your partner to offer reassurance: "Just tell me you love me." If your partner can't provide it, consider kicking him to the curb or building a more solid relationship before bringing in a third.

Embrace mistakes

Even if you try your best, you will probably screw up. There's no way to completely error-proof a threesome. But, a snafu that opens a pain tornado doesn't mean the whole experience is a bust. Crawling out of a lifelong pattern of monogamy and social programming is going to be uncomfortable at first and it's going to involve some trial and error. So, welcome your mistakes as scrumptious learning opportunities. Use them in a constructive way: investigate what went wrong, don't blame, take responsibility, be grateful for the foul-up, and do your best to avoid it next time.

> If you go into a three-or-moresome with rigid expectations, intent upon fulfilling your preconceptions exactly like the two-dimensional people in your head, this kind of defeats the purpose of doing something new and unique. Relax, explore, have fun. If it's a pleasant encounter, then you're doing okay.
>
> —Anthony Ravenscroft, Polyamory: A Roadmap for the Clueless & Hopeful

GO FOR IT!

Now, if you've decided to go for it, stop second-guessing yourself. Put the what-ifs to rest. You've done your homework, you've checked in with yourself, you know your limits, and you've communicated honestly with your partner. Pat yourself on the back. Banish doubt about yourself and your lover. Trust each other to stick to the limits. You're confident, sexy, and ready for some hot three-way lovin'. Go for it. Don't be too hard on yourself. Accept that mistakes will happen, but you'll learn in the process and it will get easier if you stay self-aware and committed to open and honest communication. Okay, you've got the scoop on having a threesome without busting your relationship and you land in a sizzling three-way sex pretzel with two hotties . . . but one is a member of the same sex. Read the next chapter for advice on making the most of your first gay lovin' experience in a three-way.

COMMUNICATION EXERCISES

1. Threesome discussion for couples—spill it now . . . Use the communication tools from this section to discuss the following:

- What scares you most about a threesome?

- What turns you on most about a threesome?
- Do you both agree on whether the third would be male, female, transsexual, gay, bi, straight?
- Do you both have a particular third in mind? (a friend, coworker?)
- Discuss which third parties feel safest for both of you.

2. Assess your sex life

- How satisfied are you with your sex life? What's working? What isn't working? What do you really want when it comes to sex? Write your answers. Share them with each other.
- Tell each other your complete sexual history including how many people you've shagged and the nitty-gritty details of what you did with them. If your relationship can't weather this, a three-way isn't going to fly.
- Masturbate to orgasm in front of each other with no assistance from each other.
- Tell each other of any affairs, fantasies, or flirtations you have had since you've been together.

3. Scavenge for truth

Even if you passed the quiz with flying colors, complete the following exercises:

- Share your answers from the pre-threesome relationship quiz (below) and take the opportunity to tell each other anything you've withheld or lied about.
- Tell your partner a secret you never thought you'd reveal.
- Assess your relationship. What's working? What isn't working? What do you really want?

4. Practice your communication skills

If you're not an expert at asking for what you want and saying no, practice these skills at a cuddle party (www.cuddleparty.com). These aren't sex parties; they actually provide a comfortable, safe environment to practice honest and direct communication with strangers.

5. Take a quiz: is your relationship ready for a threesome?

Threesomes can put your relationship at risk. (But then again, so can monogamy). It's generally wisest for couples to wait at least a year to build a decent foundation together. It also helps if you're skilled at communicating openly, clearly, and quickly with each other and solving difficulties efficiently. And it's helpful if you're both already satisfied with your sex life. Take this quiz to find out:

1. Have you ever cheated on your partner but never told him? (N-1)
2. Have you ever cheated on your partner but told her immediately? (Y-1)
3. Have you been together more than one year? (Y-1)
4. Have you told your partner any deeply guarded secrets about yourself? (Y-1)
4. Do you feel like you can "be yourself" around your partner? (Y-1)
5. Does your partner know how to please you in bed? (Y-1)
6. Is there anything you'd like in bed that you haven't asked for? (N-1)
7. Do you have any sexual fantasies that you haven't told your partner? (N-1)
8. Do you fake orgasms with your partner? (N-2)
9. Is there anything important you've withheld from your partner? (N-4. There always is).
10. Do you feel that your relationship is strong and committed? (Y-1)
11. Do you feel confident that your relationship could endure tough times? (Y-1)
12. Are you confident that your partner has not had a secret affair? (Y-1)
13. Do you feel your partner understands you

when you're discussing difficult topics or issues you don't agree on? (Y-1)

12–14 points: Your relationship is in a solid place for a threesome. You've gotten some basic communication skills down and you can probably handle the extra challenge.

9–11 points: Your relationship is in a decent place for a threesome. Put in some work clearing up any past lies and work on your communication skills.

6–8 points: Your relationship isn't exactly a model of open communication and honesty. You might be able to prepare for a threesome, but it's going to take a big commitment and lots of work.

0–5 points: Your relationship is already on the rocks. Don't muddy the waters with another set of arms.

6. Complete a threesome checklist

- Do you feel that you have made your own decision regarding threesome participation?___
- Have you developed code words for communicating?__
- Do you feel that you expressed yourself clearly and honestly?__

- Do you feel that your partner has expressed herself clearly and honestly?___
- Have you agreed on limits that feel acceptable to you?__
- Do you trust your partner to uphold the limits you've established? ____
- Are you both committed to communicating honestly, directly, and openly about whatever emotions arise during and after the threesome?__

CHAPTER 5

DISCOVERING THE INNER QUEER: WHAT TO DO WHEN SAME-SEX LOVIN' IS PART OF THE EQUATION

> To interrogate oneself tirelessly on one's sexual drives seems to me self-destructive. One can be aroused, for example, by the sight of a holly leaf, an apple tree, or a male cardinal bird on a spring morning. As deeply rooted as they are in our sentimental and erotic lives, we must consider that our genitals can be quite thoughtless.
>
> —John Cheever

My first threesome fantasies didn't raise any disturbing questions. Talking dirty with my husband about a threesome with another woman was just good, clean fun. My sexual identity was clear-cut: I was an open-minded, heterosexual woman indulging in a classic, all-American fantasy. But when we actually brought another chick into the bedroom and the smell of her neck nearly made me come, things started to get fuzzy. In fantasyland, gay was great, but when I actually experienced same-sex attraction, it was more unsettling than I expected. I was way gayer than I had ever imagined, but I wasn't sure what exactly that meant. Was I gay deep down? Would I have to permanently turn in my straight card? Maybe I was just an L.I.T. (lesbian in threesomes)?

Given the basic math, even threesomes with three self-identified straight people include at least some homoerotic potential. For me, the same-sex attraction in a threesome catalyzed a sexual identity crisis. As an obsessive researcher, I had to get to the bottom of it all and fast. A cocktail of shame and fear surfaced and I knew that denial wasn't going to work. So, I went on an investigative quest to understand and quantify my own gayness; I set out to determine whether the mind-melting hotness of this threesome was "normal" or if it meant that I was a dyke to the core. I isolated the variables: I slept with butches, bi femmes, lesbian femmes, and various combinations of three. Sometimes it was hot, sometimes it wasn't.

The data crunching revealed that my turn-on couldn't be catalogued according to simple gender formulas. I found myself undeniably bewitched, dazzled, and smitten by some men *and* some women. Desire proved to be more nuanced, slippery, capricious, and shape-shifting than network T.V. had led me to believe. I discovered a magnificent gray area with unexpected twists and turns. And even if Americans wish sexuality could easily fit into neat categories, it's just not possible for everyone—it certainly isn't for me. For some, a gay or straight identity fits snugly like a square peg in a square hole; for others, those identities leave something out. Between the poles of 100 percent gay and 100 percent straight, there's a complex landscape with a vast range of emotions, sexual feelings, and sensual expressions. And knowing that sexuality can be more complex than conventional identity labels suggest, might allow us the freedom to explore a sumptuous panoply of erotic and emotional possibilities. Do I identify as bisexual now? Well, sure, but I also identify as trisexual, pansexual, pervert extraordinaire, and queer. I definitely don't call myself "straight."

Threesomes offer an ideal opportunity to explore bisexuality with a built-in hetero safety net. If you're going to swing it three-way style, you'll have to get in touch with your inner queer. And finding that inner queer is much easier when you understand the social, emotional, and sexual dimensions of same-sex threesome action. Then, it's up to you to figure out how far you're willing to go.

> Sexuality is something that surprises us and takes us places we didn't expect to go. Why else does psychoanalysis spend so much time delving into desire and sexual identity?
>
> —Kenji Yoshino, law professor, Yale University

CONSIDER THE CONTINUUM

In the late 1940s and 1950s, American sex researcher Alfred Kinsey popularized the notion of a sexual continuum (zero to six) ranging from exclusive straightness (zero) to exclusive gayness (six). Kinsey researched more than eighteen thousand men and women on their sexual behavior and found that even during that sexually conservative era, many Americans were actually having sexual experiences that sharply contrasted with publicly held norms. Finding that 50 percent of the men he interviewed acknowledged erotic responses to their own sex, Kinsey concluded that most adults harbor some bisexual impulses.

> Males do not represent two discrete populations, heterosexual and homosexual. The world is not to be divided into sheep and goats. It is a fundamental of

taxonomy that nature rarely deals with discrete categories. . . . The living world is a continuum in each and every one of its aspects.

—American sexologist Alfred Kinsey

VOCABULARY BUILDER

Innate bisexuality

Sigmund Freud introduced the term, meaning that all humans are born with bisexual impulses. In Freud's estimation, all humans are bisexual to some extent, but learn to constrain those impulses to fit socially accepted sexual norms. (Freud also characterized humans as "polymorphous perverse," meaning having the innate ability to find nearly any object a source of erotic fascination and fulfillment.)

While many Americans are familiar with the concept of the sexual continuum popularized by Kinsey, for the most part, mainstream society still assumes that there are only two discrete sexual identities (straight and gay). Even while Bay-area hipsters indulge in an endless smorgasbord of sexual identities (from polyamorous to pansexual), mainstream society still endorses a simple gay-straight binary. Americans seem to prefer clear-cut sexual identities: are you gay or straight? And bisexuality is often written off as a cop-out for those too chicken to own up to their "real" gayness. These "tourists" or "fence-sitters" are criticized for privately reaping the benefits of gay sex without sacrificing the social advantages of heterosexual privilege. A *New York Times* article, titled "Straight, Gay, or Lying?" (July 5, 2005) suggested that a recent study showed that self-proclaimed bisexuals are actually just full of shit. And, bisexuals often carry a stigma in the gay community as "experimenters" and heartbreakers, who ultimately return to a straight lifestyle. The underlying assumption: bisexuality is just a temporary pit stop between "real" identities of gay and straight. Or, as Samantha on *Sex and the City* put it, "a layover on the way to Gaytown." That's poppycock.

Clearly, there's still some major cultural discomfort around bisexuality. In an article for *Stanford Law Review,* Yale legal scholar Kenji Yoshino argued that gays and straights have "erased" bisexuality—pretended that it doesn't exist for various cultural and political reasons.[6]

Ultimately, bisexuality could become just another sexual identity label or it could serve to unravel sexual orientation as a category and challenge us to think beyond labels. There are so many ways of distinguishing between people on the basis of sexuality. We could choose to distinguish people on the basis of whether they have sex a lot or a little, or whether they prefer sex with emotional connections or getting it on with strangers. So it's a bit curious why the biological sexes of the people schtooping has become the central way of thinking about sexuality.

> I would say that I am truly bisexual—I have no preference for gender. In fact, I typically describe myself as gender-blind, because I tend to notice everything else about someone before I spot that they are male or female. "Oh, you have blue eyes, and a mohawk, and you like theater, and you're training to be a veterinarian. Oh, and you're a female." I tend to be much more attracted to energy or personality than physical form.
>
> —Sue, 35

Sexuality may be too complex to be neatly packaged into two (or even three) labels. And, in the post-identity era, the concept of sexual fluidity seems to be inching toward the mainstream. Some radical hipsters and Gen Yers, who embrace a sliding scale model of sexuality over outdated identity labels, prefer to be called fluid, pansexual, or to avoid labels altogether. These labels express an acceptance of all gender possibilities (including those who don't fit into the gender binary) and call attention to the idea that sexual identity is merely a social construct. These postmodern lovers argue that attraction doesn't fit neatly into categories. By dropping labels, we may be more open to experiencing and relishing the mysterious ways that sexuality morphs, expands, and shifts over a lifetime. By letting go of stone-carved identities, it's much easier to follow sparkly connections in the moment, wherever they appear. One twenty-four-year-old female college student put it this way:

> In America few people understand the fluidity of gender and sexuality. People are still caught in this fucking binary—you're a man or you're a woman, you're straight or you're gay. They don't understand that there are many shades of gray. People need to understand that just because you're a flaming heterosexual man, that doesn't mean you don't enjoy sucking cock every now and then. When you get away from the stigma of, "if I suck cock, I'm gay and that's bad," you can start enjoying yourself. If I have to label myself, I say I'm "queer" rather than "bisexual"" because it's a more fluid label. Fuck all the binary sexual identities.

I believe that every single human is born with a potential for bisexual response. The real mystery is why anyone would be exclusively heterosexual or exclusively homosexual. My ideal universe is one in which people have a primary sexual orientation but feel absolutely free to experiment across gender lines, to respond to the moment, to the person. That's sophisticated! That's truly creative!

—Camille Paglia, American social critic

My feeling is that labels are for canned food. . . . I am what I am—and I know what I am.

—R.E.M.'s Michael Stipe, discussing "the whole queer-straight-bi thing" in *Rolling Stone*

VOCABULARY BUILDER

Heteroflexible

Kind of straight . . . but reserving the right to fuck anyone.

Even today, with gay pride rainbows adorning urban storefronts and radical hipsters flaunting "pansexual" identities, many self-proclaimed "straight" Americans dabbling in gay sex for the first time still contend with shame, guilt, and fear. Considering that homophobia still looms large in our society, it's no wonder that so many people who get turned on by same-sex action continue to identify as "straight." Many people who occasionally get off with someone of the same sex just aren't willing to ditch their "straight" identity labels. (The best-selling *The Straight Girl's Guide to Sleeping with Chicks* sums up this position.) And many women who aren't into "raw sex" with other women in one-on-one scenarios, find themselves super turned on by women in three-ways. Sometimes, threesomes offer a way to experience same-sex attraction without having to directly confront our own homophobia. My first girlfriend and I felt way more comfortable fucking when there was a man in the room, even if he wasn't involved in the action, because it felt much straighter. We were both self-identified "straight" women, who happened to be getting turned on by same-sex action, but we were both confused and ashamed, which made the experience a whole lot less wonderful. So, if it makes you feel better to call yourself straight while you're having gay sex, go for it. Whether you decide to use a "straight," "gay," or "bi" label is up to you, but don't let shame and fear block your bliss. If you can let go of the labels and be open to the particular hotness of the moment, you may have much more fun getting your same-sex groove on in a threesome.

Why Do All These Homosexuals Keep Sucking My Cock?

Look, I'm not a hateful person or anything—I believe we should all live and let live. But lately, I've been having a real problem with these homosexuals. You see, just about wherever I go these days, one of them approaches me and starts sucking my cock.

—Bruce Heffernan, *The Onion,* October 28, 1998

VOCABULARY BUILDER

Pansexuality

A step beyond bisexual, referring to an all-inclusive sexual orientation which includes people who don't fit into the gender binary of male-female. Sometimes described as the ability to get the hots for someone regardless of gender. In the hit TV show, *Will & Grace,* Karen Walker's pastry chef (who had sex with Will, Karen, and Rosario) described himself as "pansexual."

LESSONS FROM HISTORY

Americans haven't always understood sexuality in terms of gay and straight identities. Before the binary gay-straight structure dominated the way Americans think about sexuality, a world of more diverse sexual options reigned. Long before Stonewall put gay identity on the map, working-class men had sex with other men in a hopping, guy-centric nightlife in turn-of-the-century New York City.[7] And, while these men engaged in guy-on-guy sexual contact, they weren't conceptualized as homosexuals; instead, the term referred to practices, rather than identity. Turn-of-the-century sexual identities were defined by gender roles enacted during sex, rather than the choice of male or female sex partners. In other words, men who performed the "active" (or "male") role in sex with other men weren't considered gay, while men who performed the "passive" (or "female") role in sex with men were labeled effeminate "fairies."

The term *homosexual* was originally used in Europe and was first introduced in English by German psychiatrist and sex researcher Richard von Krafft-Ebing in his compendium of sexual research titled *Psychopathalia Sexualis (1892)*.

White House Kink

In *The Intimate World of Abraham Lincoln* (2004), psychologist and sex researcher, C. A. Tripp, argues that Abe Lincoln was gay. Honest Abe had a rocky marriage, slept in a twin bed with a male friend for years and wrote passionate letters to his guy pals. While today two men incidentally bumping elbows on the street looks a little queer, men in nineteenth century America commonly slept in bed together, snuggled all night and wrote each other deeply intimate letters. And, no one snickered because this kind of intimacy between men was entirely acceptable, standard fare at the time. And, since nineteenth-century Americans didn't even have a vocabulary for same-sex love (the term "homosexual" wasn't even coined until the late 1800s), historians have a helluva time trying to figure out who was involved in common intimate male friendships and who was getting bona fide gay sex. The verdict is still out on whether Honest Abe actually got frisky with the gents in his bed, but regardless of whether he took it up the Hershey highway, Lincoln's letters prove that he loved men and some loved him back.

And, in Victorian America, college girls routinely had "crushes" on each other—they shared twin beds, wrote each other love letters and shared passionately romantic intimacy. In *The Way We Never Were*, historian Stephanie Coontz noted:

> Perfectly respectable Victorian women wrote to each other in terms such as these: "I hope for you so much, and feel so eager for you . . . that the expectation once more to see your face again, makes me feel hot and feverish." They recorded the "furnace blast" of their "passionate attachments" to each other. . . . They carved their initials into trees, set flowers in front of one another's portraits, danced together, kissed, held hands, and endured intense jealousies over rivals or small slights.[8]

Although women weren't encouraged to choose these female relationships over heterosexual marriage, these intense "romantic friendships" between women were considered natural in Victorian America and only became stigmatized and pathologized in the early twentieth century, after sexologists defined "lesbianism" and subsequently identified it as a medical malady. Some contemporary historians have argued that the Victorians, who have been stereotyped as the epitome of prudishness, in some ways allowed more latitude in terms of sexual diversity and expression than contemporary America. A look at the Victorians shows that sexual orientation is not a fixed, timeless, or objective way to understand sexuality. And this historical perspective can inspire us to expand contemporary notions of sexuality so that we may move more freely across a broad spectrum of sexual behaviors, preferences, and attractions.

> This history shows clearly that to develop gay and lesbian politics solely around the concept of a fixed identity is problematic, for it requires the drawing of static and arbitrary boundaries in a situation that is fluid and changing. The challenge we face—to organize a movement that both defends gay rights in a homophobic society on the basis of the assumption of a fixed gay identity, and envisions a society where sexuality is not polarized into fixed homo/hetero identities—is difficult but worthwhile.
>
> —Historians Elizabeth Kennedy
> and Madeline Davis,
> *Boots of Leather, Slippers of Gold*

VOCABULARY BUILDERS

The doll racket

A term for lesbianism in the 1940s

Usage: "I'm in the doll racket, baby."

Tribadism

Derived from the ancient Greek word tribein, meaning "to rub." Female-to-female genital sex or genital rubbing. A.k.a. bumping fur, scissoring, polishing mirrors, and making tortillas.

Smashing

A term used in Victorian America to describe two adolescent girls developing an intimate, passionate relationship with each other.

Famous Historical Figures Who Slept with Both Men and Women

Alexander the Great

Janis Joplin

Sandra Bernhardt

Virginia Woolf

Julius Caesar

1990s rockstar Kurt Cobain

Spiritual leader Ram Das

Poet Edna St. Vincent Millay

Madonna

Courtney Love

Socrates

Marlon Brando

Tennis star Martina Navratilova

Georgia O'Keeffe

Mexican painter Frieda Kahlo

D. H. Lawrence

Preeminent anthropologist Margaret Mead

Mick Jagger

American playwright and novelist Gore Vidal

Erotica writer Anaïs Nin

VOCABULARY BUILDER

Bi-curious

A term commonly found in personal ads, suggesting an interest in same-sex "experimentation."

GIRL-ON-GIRL

Today it's common for straight women to sexually experiment with other women. Sorority girls do it. Middle-aged swingers do it. Madonna does it. And just about every college chick in America has tried it. And, for some reason, when women dyke out, they aren't suspected of being gay or even bisexual—they're just considered sexy. Female bisexuality has become mainstream chic and trendy probably in part because it fulfills a straight male fantasy. Girl-on-girl booty just ups a straight woman's fuckability quotient and reaffirms her position as an object of male fantasy. The women-as-sex-object element of these lesbian performances may irk some feminists and card-carrying lesbians and bisexuals; while others consider these displays a way for women to reclaim their sexual agency and the freedom to pursue sexual desire however it arises. These days, even self-proclaimed straight women can relish the joys of gay sex. And, take it from me: chicks are hot, give it a try.

Tales from the Trenches: Girl-on-Girl Lovin'

I've been in lots of threesomes with straight women, whose pussies I've licked during a threesome with my boyfriend, but they never did anything back to me. They just weren't hot for me and I got sick of feeling like the evil molester. Then my boyfriend and I were seduced by a lesbian. That was the first time I had a threesome with a woman who wasn't straight; she was someone who actually enjoyed my body. She made me feel beautiful and great about lesbian sex. That was amazing!

—Eileen, 25

We've picked up women for threesomes who have never messed around with women before, and suddenly, they want to try it because it's hip and cool for everyone to test their bisexuality. Sometimes they get halfway through and think, *Wow, this wasn't what I expected.* You can see it in their eyes. Of course, sometimes they get in there and love it, and it's the greatest thing ever.

—Phillip, 27

I've been in various monogamous, polyamorous, and "open" relationships with men and women. I was once in a long-term threesome relationship with two men, all of us being bisexual. I was also in a monogamous relationship with a woman that lasted for several years. Many people assumed at that point that I had become a lesbian. It just happened that our energies clicked, regardless of gender. People need to label relationships for some reason, rather than just letting them be as they are.

—Erin, 36

Another benefit of sleeping with women is that it's easier to trade the dominant sexual position back and forth, whereas when sleeping with men it can be a little tougher. With women, since there aren't any social gender roles establishing how bedroom dynamics should play out, and there's no cock, the dominant position is entirely up for grabs. This can be incredibly fun, surprising, and challenging.

—Maggie, 28

Kobe antelope engage in female-on-female mounting sessions and lick each other's vulvas.

BOY-ON-BOY BOOTY

> Every straight guy should have a man's tongue in his mouth at least once.
>
> —Madonna

While many straight women may not hesitate much before shagging women, straight American guys tend to be more paranoid about having guy-on-guy sexual contact. In America sexual contact between men is still stigmatized, and there isn't much acceptance of sexual fluidity for men. American cultural logic seems to suggest that being a manly man means fucking women. But while the mere thought of kissing a man makes many straight American guys bristle, European guys don't have this knee-jerk homophobic reaction. Gay shame isn't cross-cultural. Many countries around the world are more permissive when it comes to male-to-male affection and sexual behavior: in 1997, half of adult male university students in Sri Lanka reported having their first sexual experiences with men, and Scandinavian countries are famous for their progressive ways when it comes to male sexuality. One "fluid" twenty-eight-year-old man, who grew up in Germany, explains how European sexual mores shaped his ability to explore sexuality freely:

> I'm really lucky because I didn't grow up with any these issues. Germany is extremely sexually liberated—porn is shown on their regular channels after eight PM, kids look at nudie magazines. Homosexual behavior is really no big deal there, so I ended up sexually interacting with men first. None of us considered ourselves gay; in fact, we all had massive crushes on female classmates, but we got sexual gratification from each other at a young age, so I never had any hang-ups with having sex with men. At this point, I wouldn't sleep with a man on my own. After having tried out everything there is and having had lots of men in my bed, it's pretty obvious that I'm primarily attracted to women. I've recently gotten together with a male/female couple—that's when I realized I've had a very strong desire and fantasy for over a decade to be with a man and a woman simultaneously. There's something incredibly intense when three people are involved with each other sexually and emotionally.

Getting over the shakes: first-time gay love in threesomes

For those lacking a gay sex résumé, here's some advice for your first threesome with someone of the same sex:

Ask Sally Threesome

Q: My girlfriend wants to have a threesome with a bi guy. I'm nervous about having a dude in the room.

A: If you're really not into it, don't be pressured into it. But it wouldn't hurt to consider pushing your boundaries. How do you feel about having a threesome with another guy if you've agreed not to touch each other? Remember, *heteroflexibility* is the buzzword these days. Sexual orientation just isn't black-and-white. There's a huge gray area between 100 percent straight and 100 percent gay. And many people fall somewhere in between. So just because you get a wicked hot blowjob from a guy doesn't mean you have to declare yourself a flaming pillow-biter for life. And men who are comfortable enough with their sexuality to dabble in same-sex exploration without spiraling into a homophobic tailspin win extra hotness points with the ladies. Plus, what doesn't kill you makes you stronger.

Try a vee. If the thought of being in the same room as another erect penis gives you the willies, don't despair. A threesome can be an ideal opportunity to explore your voyeuristic or exhibitionist side. (Or, if you're a guy, make the threesome all about pleasing the woman.) Vees are essentially threesomes with two people who are attracted to a third person, but not to each other. If a vee sounds like a safe way to have a sexual experience with another guy, make sure to enlist a straight guy as your three-way buddy. Knowing that the other guy is straight might help you relax and enjoy. And if you end up cozying up to the guy a bit more than you expected, great. Even if you don't even make eye contact with the other guy, at least it might give you a nonthreatening opportunity to warm up to the idea. And, who knows, maybe your next three-way will include a guy-on-guy elbow contact. Wow. Some straight guys even prefer M^2F threesomes to threesomes with two women because there's less pressure or because they offer voyeuristic bliss.

> I've had two threesomes, one with a guy and a woman, another with two women. Actually, even though having two women is the typical straight male fantasy, I actually enjoyed the one with a guy and a woman much better. I'm straight and the other guy was straight, so that wasn't an issue. But, with the two women, they were both straight and weren't into each other, so I felt like the host and I felt like there wasn't enough of me to go around.
>
> —Phil, 37

> I wasn't in a threesome with another guy until I was thirty or so. I've made it alone with a man maybe half a dozen times. I've gone down on a guy, I can do it, but there's no affection, it's just tactile. Normally I fuck them, they don't fuck me. I don't even like a finger up my ass. Now I prefer a threesome of two strongly sexed heterosexual men and a girl. It's more visual. She's warm and moist, and I watch his cock slide in and out and identify—it's like fucking twice. If I do get freaky with the guy, I'll fuck him and come on his face. I still want the girl to get him off.
>
> —Male respondent to a sociological threesome study by Arno Karlen, *Threesomes: Studies in Sex, Power, and Intimacy*

Recruit a female ringleader for M²F threesomes. If you're a guy in a relationship with a woman, ask her how she feels about you making out with a guy. If she's into it, ask her to lead the way. Having a female ringleader to catalyze your first guy-on-guy encounter can ease the process. If she tells you it turns her on to watch you kiss another guy, the scenario might be less likely to threaten your sexual identity or masculinity. Some women find watching male-on-male lovin' a major turn-on: "I find men who are so comfortable with their sexuality incredibly sexy. When a man can express raw sexual passion for another guy and not worry about it diminishing his masculinity, I'm impressed. There's nothing like seeing two men kissing." Another woman described her thrill at watching her husband make out with another guy:

> My husband was being flirty with this guy. They're both totally straight guys, so I was impressed. We

Tales from the Trenches: My First Time with Another Guy

The first time my girlfriend and I fooled around with a guy, he and I didn't touch much, and afterward I was all pissed off because I was convinced he was "using" me to get to her. In other words, I thought he didn't really like me, but did want to have sex with my girlfriend and therefore tolerated my presence. Part of it was that I'm naturally jealous of my girlfriend (I mean, come on, she's like twice as hot as me), and part was my own homophobia. Had he been a she, I'm sure I would have just jumped on him and seen what happened, but since he was a he, I didn't want to risk being rejected by a guy. Heaven forbid I was "bi" and he wasn't. As open as I am (I honestly don't give a shit what other people's orientations are, and in fact respect people more for being adventurous) I still have my own hang-ups about my bisexuality.

Anyway, my girlfriend told the guy about it, and he said he had avoided touching me for similar reasons—he was afraid I wasn't really bi and didn't want him to touch me. Welcome to homophobia. One night we all talked about it together, resolved the issue, had a few drinks, dressed my girlfriend up in latex, and had a fucking blast.

I'm actually much happier with my perception of my

all went dancing. My husband put me between him and this other guy, then they started kissing over my shoulder. I was like, "Oh, my god, my husband is kissing a man!" They started grabbing, kissing, and molesting me, and I happily acquiesced. We ended up in the bedroom, rolling around and having a hot threesome.

sexuality now. I feel like "Yes. I am bi, and I like fooling around with men every now and then." It's almost like a point of pride, although I admit I don't tell most people. I'm sure my folks wouldn't care, but I haven't told them yet. At the same time, I had a really good time flirting and dancing with a British cross-dresser the other night. I don't think I would have been comfortable doing that before having the threesome with a guy.

I also like the fact that when people talk shit about gay or bi men I can be "Fuck you, I'm bi, do you have a problem with me?" It seems to be such a gut reaction in this country to make fun of gay people, even if you don't really have a problem with them. I have to admit I do it, too, sometimes (although only when it's funny).

So, the first time I was pretty uncomfortable because I didn't know what the boundaries were. While it's fine to say we should have outlined them ahead of time, that's hard to do when you're drunk and in the heat of the moment. By talking about what hadn't worked afterward, we were able to have a much better experience the second time.

As for what we did, the guy and I only did oral (the second time) and both of us had sex with my girlfriend. It was great at the time, and I haven't felt bad about it since, as in "Oh, my God, I've sucked cock!" However, I've never been one to much care about what society thinks of me. Still, most of my friends don't know. I reckon I need to work on that.

—Clint, 33

Enlist a gay guide. Sleeping with straight people (who have their own shame and homophobia to deal with) may exacerbate your own fears about gay sex. While self-identified "straight" people may find themselves turned on by same-sex action in athreesome, they're likely to have their own shame and fear about gay sexuality. And, if you're not comfortably bisexual or gay, sleeping with self-identified straight people can multiply your own fears.

So if you've never even kissed another guy, but you're curious, consider enlisting an openly gay or bisexual guy to show you the ropes. There's nothing like sleeping with gay or bisexual people who are comfortable with their sexuality. Plus, that way, you can just sit back and let your gay guide please you. If you subscribe to the "a mouth is a mouth" philosophy, you should have no trouble enjoying yourself. Maybe you'll even get so turned on that you'll gladly return the favor. Even if the encounter raises scary sexual-identity questions for you, having a proud gay guide initiate you into the joys of gay sex may facilitate a smoother journey.

TEST YOUR GAYNESS

As a result of a 1980 study in *Penthouse Forum* magazine, American sex researcher and psychiatrist Fritz Klein developed a sexual orientation grid to evaluate sexuality. Klein suggested that sexual orientation was comprised of various, fluid factors that changed over time. Take the quiz to investigate your own sexual proclivities. If nothing else, the grid might clarify just how complex sexual orientation can be.

Using a scale from 1 (exclusively heterosexual) to 7 (exclusively homosexual), rate your preference for each variable on the grid.

	PAST	PRESENT	IDEAL
1. Sexual attraction To whom are you sexually attracted?			
2. Sexual behavior Who do you have sex with primarily?			
3. Sexual fantasies About whom are your sexual fantasies?			
4. Emotional preference Are you emotionally closest to members of the opposite or same sex?			
5. Social preference Do you prefer to spend most of your time with same-sex friends or opposite-sex friends?			
6. Total (add scores from each column)			
7. Determine your past, present, and ideal sexual orientation (divide each total by 5)			

GAY LOVIN' 101

You've been socially conditioned to be straight. And maybe you'll find you are 100 percent straight, but if you've never been with someone of the same sex, there's no way to know for sure. You'll probably have the best time if you stop obsessing about what it all means in terms of sexual identity and explore what feels good to you. Instead of diving in all at once, start slow with some kissing, cuddling, and hugging. Escalate if you get turned on. If you find that it just isn't your bag, no big deal. At least you tried something new. If you find that you like it, you'll be glad you didn't miss out.

There are lots of preconceptions and fears about same-sex action in a threesome, so check out these tips before taking the plunge:

Don't be competitive

You might have a dazzling nipple-licking technique, but don't expect to be the best at everything. Many women and men fear their sexual prowess won't match up in a threesome. Relax, you might learn something. One confident green-eyed beauty said, "My friend gives the best blow jobs in the world. She knows how to get the whole thing down her throat and she does this swirl thing with her tongue. So, I let her blow my boyfriend. She's a friend, and I knew she was really good at it, so I wanted my boyfriend to experience that. Plus, I learned a few things from watching her."

Love what you've got

Men considering threesomes with other guys worry their cocks will be smaller or abs flabbier, and women considering threesomes with other women report similar fears. Most of us know that the media tell us our bodies are imperfect—too fat, too smelly, too wrinkled, or too soft. And, even though we may know it's horseshit, these messages still seep into our brains and mess with our self-esteem. In a media-saturated country where most images of women and men have been photoshopped to perfection, it's hard to find a living supermodel (much less a computer programmer), who doesn't wish she had sexier earlobes or a tighter ass. So, buck up, even the prettiest bombshell has body insecurities. You can spend your life thinking your butt's too big (or your cock's too small) or feeling sexy as hell. Make the choice to appreciate your body as it is. Physical insecurities can wreck a potentially dreamy threesome.

Don't expect to be an instant expert

Don't expect to be an instant expert at handling pussy or cock just because you have one. Maybe you haven't paid attention to what feels good on you. Learning how to please someone of the same sex takes some trial and error. Don't be embarrassed about not being a pro, and remember, a willingness to learn is always charming.

Pussies are yummy

Many women grow up with shame about the way their pussies look, smell, or taste. The barrage of "freshness" commercials and tuna jokes can make women fear that their pussies are unappetizing. (Cocks, for some reason, don't get such a bad rap . . . in spite of their excretions.) While some women have realized this is bullshit, others still believe their kitties smell bad. Not only does this myth dampen the pleasure for women receiving oral sex, but it also makes women tepid about going down on other women. Performing oral sex on a woman and finding that it's not disgusting can be a fabulous way to get over any shame you have about your own body. You might even find yourself getting turned on in the process. One woman explained her recent revelation with eating pussy: "My boyfriend used to beg me for threesomes with another woman and tell me stories about me going down on another woman. I just couldn't imagine doing it in real life because I thought pussies were so gross—that was until I tried it. I found the smell and taste intoxicating; it was a major turn-on." Pussy may or may not do it for you, but there's only one way to find out.

TIPS FOR HANDLING PUSSY

Take your time

If you're used to sleeping with men, you might be used to going straight for the cock. This works for guys, but clits require patience. So, don't go for direct stimulation right away. Discover what body parts she likes having touched. Go slowly. Start by lightly touching, kissing, biting, and licking her all over. Teasing can be very delicious. Start with a hot breath and light touch on her neck, arms, and hips. Lick her. Smell her and let her know how much you enjoy the feel of her skin. Discover and savor her inner elbow, her earlobe. As she's getting more turned on, start touching her pussy, and keep touching other body parts: lick her nipples, grab her ass, and stroke her thighs. Basically, get her to the point where she's dying for you to tickle her button.

Watch, listen, and, when in doubt ask

The most important thing to remember is that everyone likes something different. Sure, it helps to have a bag of tricks to try and then explore what works for each person. Remember that different sensations will feel good at different stages in her turn-on, so pay attention. Watch for clues. If she suddenly jolts or quivers, you're applying too much pressure, so back off a bit. Watch for feedback: moans, breath changes, body movement, sighs, and other clues. Let her responses guide your pressure and techniques. If you're not sure, ask. Don't ask generic questions like, Are you okay? Instead, ask specific questions like: Faster? Slower? Harder? Softer? Side to side? Circles? Do you want me to hold still for a minute? Tell me when to start again. Do you want me to keep going just like this?

Familiarize yourself with the territory

Note the location of the clitoris, the sweet spot, where millions of nerves bundle together to maximize pleasure. It's much bigger than you'd think. It actually has "legs," which come down on both sides under the inner lips.

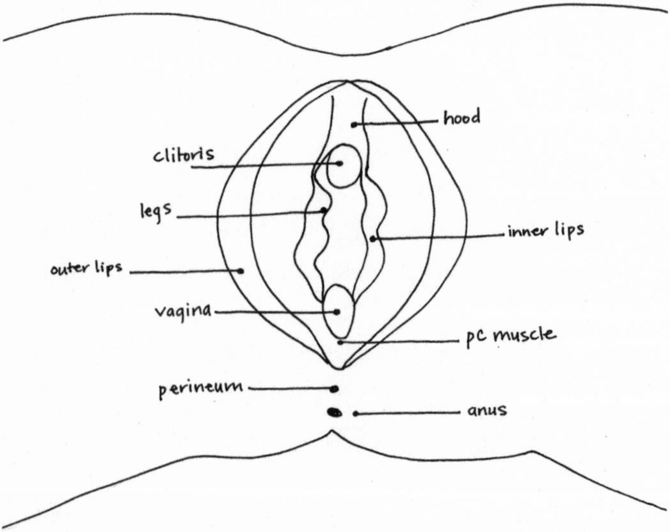

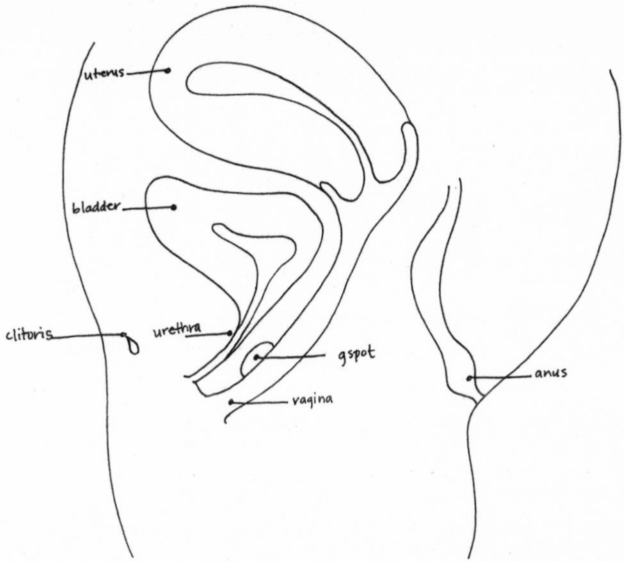

Searching for orgasms

Women's sexual rhythm and pacing is different from men's, so that's a delectable new experience. Build in waves, rather than building directly toward an orgasm; it's hotter to build, then back off, build, then back off. Some women find that penetration competes with clitoral stimulation and pulls focus, moving them away from orgasm, so they need lighter penetration at first. Others find that penetration helps orgasm build. Change techniques at the beginning of arousal, but then as she gets closer to orgasm, stick with one move until she comes.

Stick your hand down her pants

Notice what feels good when you masturbate, then try those tricks on her. A few basic hand techniques for beginners:

- Put whole hand on top of her mound and tap it gently.
- Pinch the hood and rock your fingers, without touching the clit.
- Massage or tug at outer lips.
- Gently run your fingers up and down between the inner and outer lips.
- When her legs are closed, gently pinch her lips closed with your fingers.
- Lightly stroke her outer lips and tug at them gently.

> The most direct route to pussy: nipples. Nipples produce a love hormone that can get women seriously worked up—try licking, sucking, pinching. Don't underestimate nipple play.

Eating pussy

If you're still worried that you're not going to like the smell or taste down there, start slow. Smell her skin; kiss her inner thigh; enjoy it. Gently run your lips over her underwear. How does she smell? Rub her mound with your hand, try a taste of her on your fingers. Another trick: try showering together or taking a bath together before getting into it.

One way to be a good lover is to alleviate her fears about receiving oral sex. Many women fear their lovers aren't enjoying giving them head, that their pussies don't smell sweet or that they'll take too long to cum. These worries can kill the turn-on. One way to be a stellar lover is to defuse the common fears women have about receiving it. There's nothing hotter than making it very clear how much you enjoy the smell and taste of her box. If you're enjoying it, let her know. This is especially true in a threesome, where many women fear that the other woman involved is doing it as a show for the guy and that she doesn't really enjoy it. Tell her how wet you're getting. Put her hand on your pussy, so she can feel how wet you are from going down on her.

Pussy eating is largely about pressure and pacing. Go slow and change the pressure based on her responses. Lick and kiss everything but her clit for a long time. Let that be the final treat, after she's been getting turned on for a while. A few moves that may leave her smiling:

- Start by lightly kissing her outer lips.
- Using a soft, flat tongue, very slowly lick up toward her clit, stopping just before the clit.

- Slowly run your tongue along the area between her outer and inner lips.
- Keep touching other body parts. Lick and squeeze her nipples.
- When she's very turned on, place your index fingers and thumbs in a diamond shape around her lips to gently hold them open.
- Slowly circle her clit with your tongue. Don't hit the clit directly.
- Experiment with using your tongue in different ways—soft, pointy, flat, firm, and focused.
- Gently push her clit side to side or up and down.
- Use your tongue to write the alphabet on her clit.
- Lay off her clit. Clits can be super-sensitive after an orgasm, so when she comes, get off her clit. You might be able to prolong her orgasm by slowly moving down the "legs" of the clit.

G-spot

When she's very turned on, slide one or two fingers into her pussy. Gently curve your finger toward her belly button in a "come here" move. The slightly spongy spot is the G-spot. Some women go nuts when it's touched, some don't like it at all. When it is pressed too intensely, some women feel like they have to pee. It's possible to push through this feeling (she won't actually pee), or you can lighten the pressure.

Stay focused on using your mouth, while gently trying the come-hither finger move to stimulate the G-spot. The G-spot is also the touch point for the female squirting orgasms.

Bumping fur

Rubbing pussies together is one fabulously fun part of girl sex. If you're doubtful there's any point to cock-free fucking, don't write it off 'til you try it. This can be done in various positions; try missionary style first. Slide your pussy on top of hers, then lower yourself on top of her. Grind your clits together. For more pressure, grab her ass and pull her into you. (See chapter 7 for positions.)

TIPS FOR PLAYING WITH COCK

Familiarize yourself with the territory

Notice the sensitive area under the head of the cock (which often responds well to tongue flicks). Another key feature is the prostate gland, known as the male G-spot, (which triggers sensory magnificence when pressed—that's why anal sex feels so good).

Blow jobs 101

For men new to getting it on with men, if the whole sex-with-men encounter still carries so much baggage, start slow. Shut your eyes. Take a deep breath, and let the

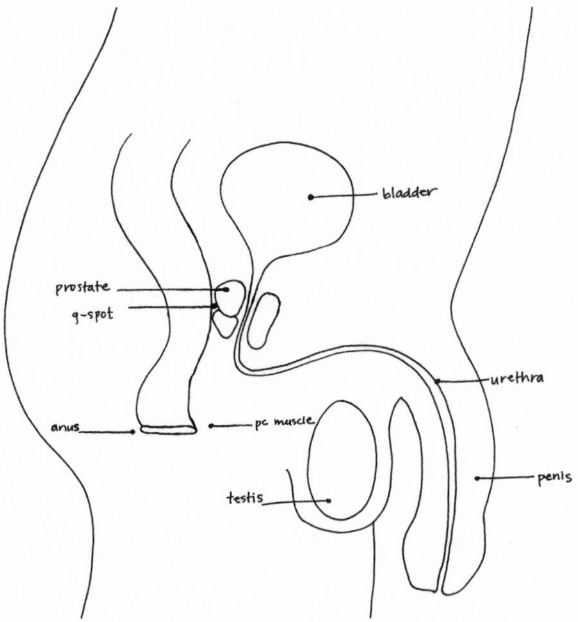

other dude go down on you first. Now, if you want to return the favor and you've never touched another cock before, try going down on him either in a 69 position or while the woman in your trio is orally pleasuring you. If someone's touching you while you're giving a blowjob, you're more likely to enjoy giving your first blowjob. There's no need to dive right in, lick around it, taste it. Go slow. Try lightly flicking on the underside of the head. Feeling ambitious? Try deep throating. If the thought of cum in your throat makes you queasy, ask your playmate to give you a warning so you can move your head.

Ass sex 101

Many guys (gay, straight, and bi) love having their asses fondled. Even straighty-pants guys get hot taking it up the Hershey highway. Enjoying ass play doesn't mean handing in your straight-guy card, so put aside sexual identity labels and experiment with what feels good. For one thing, there's a nifty little prostrate gland—sometimes called the G-spot for guys—that makes anal sex wicked hot for guys. Lots of straight guys love it when their girlfriends fuck them up the ass. Bend Over Boyfriend strap-on sales are skyrocketing. So if you've never been anally penetrated by a gal or guy, it's definitely worth a shot.

The key to backdoor booty. Lube, lube, and more lube. Assholes can't create their own lubrication, and since the lining is more fragile than the vaginal lining, artificial lube is essential for preventing tears and rips. Gel lubes work best for ass play.

Simple starter steps. Remember, anal penetration isn't easy without arousal. So start with your favorite turn-on. When you're super hard, ask your girlfriend to press the pad of a lubed-up index finger against your asshole. That way, you maintain control. Move onto her finger when you're ready. Ask her to move her finger toward the front wall of your asshole (to hit your prostate) and massage gently. If you're having fun, try taking it a step further. Ask your girlfriend to insert a small, lubed-up anal plug into your ass. How does that feel? When you're ready, ask your girlfriend to try schtooping you with a strap-on. (Sex shops make strap-on kits designed just for guys who take it in the rear from their babes.) Once you get that down, try experimenting with a guy.

PEP TALK

If the thought of brushing up against someone of the same sex still gives you the jitters, try letting go of identity labels, and consider your threesome an opportunity to explore. Sexuality comes in myriad shades of gray and you won't know where it's going to take you until you follow it. Sure, threesomes can profoundly change the way you think about your sexual identity. It can be super scary to play gay in a three-way, but it's well worth the adventure. Maybe you'll find that you love having your cock sucked by a man while your wife watches. Does that make you gay deep down? Who knows. If you don't like same-sex lovin', at least you tried; if you find that gay sex rocks your world, great, you've just doubled your pool of playmates—dive in. If you find that gay is your favorite way, then at least you didn't miss out because you were too chicken to try it. So the choice is yours—either follow that Brokeback itch and find out where it leads, or take a cold shower. . . .

Inner-queer development exercises

1. Watch gay porn.
2. Put your hand down your pants. Smell your fingers. Survive.
3. Go to a gay bar or club. Flirt with five people. Survive.
4. Ask a gay friend for a test kiss. Enjoy.

CHAPTER 6

KEEPING IT CLEAN: SAFER SEX FOR THREE

Every time I've been in a monogamous relationship, my partner has secretly cheated. And, one of them gave me an STD! When you're in a supposedly monogamous relationship, you have to pretend you're overwhelmed with passion when you cheat and that often leads people to have unprotected sex. That's why I prefer ethical nonmonogamy—it's easier to get the truth from your partners—now I trust my partners to have protected sex and to tell me if they've had unprotected sex. So, I actually feel much safer in nonmonogamous relationships.

—Christine, 35

Before getting down and dirty with three, it's super important to consider your health. There's no clear-cut way to prevent all sexually transmitted diseases—except abstinence—and where's the fun in that? But you can learn about the risks associated with different behaviors, make decisions about which risks are acceptable to you, ask your partners about their sexual histories, and make safer-sex agreements before you start getting sweaty. Here's a basic primer on diseases, how to protect yourself, how to be an ethical three-way lover, and how to prevent threesome-specific health snafus.

ETHICS, TACT, AND CLASS

You've just landed in bed with two hotties. Nothing spoils the mood like talking about all the nasties you can catch in the bedroom. Do it anyway. It's your responsibility to ask. Some seasoned ethical nonmonogamists carry their clean STD medical reports with them on dates (literally). Obviously, most sexually active Americans don't. That means you've got less to go on: whatever your lovers tell you and a visual inspection of your new lover's genitals. (A friend of mine says she always shines a bright light to inspect all cocks before she puts them anywhere near her mouth or pussy.) It would be nice to think that everyone would be perfectly forthright about their medical issues. (If you've got an STD: don't be a schmuck, fess up.) Unfortunately, many STDs are asymptomatic, and carriers don't even know they're passing a bug. So, even if you trust your new lovers to tell you the truth, unless they've been tested since their last sexual encounters (and even that might not be adequate since HIV antibodies can take up to six months to show up in lab results), there's no way to know if they're STD free. It helps to know someone's sexual history, to see a clean bill of health, to see no visible signs of infection on their nether regions, and to know STD risk factors for certain behaviors.

Safer sex personal standards and agreements

Crossing your fingers isn't the best way to protect yourself. Knowing the risks and having clear safer-sex limits will allow you to relax and enjoy smutty moments without biting your nails in the morning. Once you know the risks, make decisions about which risks you can live with. You may decide receiving unprotected oral sex is worth the risk, but ass eating isn't. Whatever you decide is your business, just make decisions about it in advance. Threesome sex can be so hot that it clouds your judgment, so it's wise to decide on safer-sex requirements in advance. Be willing to say no to sex that doesn't meet your safer-sex requirements. (Most lifestyle and erotic parties enforce strict safer-sex rules, so using condoms with this crowd won't require any arm twisting.)

To fluid bond or not to fluid bond? People in committed relationships may decide to *fluid bond,* which means taking complete STD tests and agreeing to have unprotected sex with each other. A fluid bonded couple may agree to have unprotected sex only with each other and protected sex with any third lovers; a fluid bonded threesome may agree to have unprotected sex with each other and protected sex with any other lovers. Being fluid bonded requires a lot of honesty and communication. A fluid bond works best when partners have agreed on specific safer-sex requirements for outside lovers (i.e., eating a third's pussy without a barrier may be okay, but ass eating might not). Don't pressure anyone to become fluid bonded (that can lead to dishonesty), and promise to tell each other if you "slip up" by having unprotected sex with someone else (before having sex with each other). If your partner admits to a slip-up, don't fly off the handle; be grateful for getting the truth instead of being put at risk.

VOCABULARY BUILDER

Condom commitment

An agreement to confine bodily fluid exchange and barrier-free intercourse to a closed group whose members have been screened for STDs.

THE LOWDOWN ON SEXUALLY TRANSMITTED DISEASES AND SEXUAL HEALTH

The quick and dirty

It's common knowledge that anal and vaginal intercourse have high STD transmission risks, so it's smartest to use condoms. Other items on the sexual menu carry different risks. Do your own research on your favorite activities to fully understand the risks, but here's the quick and dirty in a nutshell. Pussy-to-pussy sex carries a high risk for spreading herpes and some bacterial STDs, but a lower risk for other STDs (such as HIV). Opinions differ on whether unprotected oral sex is worth the risks. Some STDs (such as herpes) and bacterial STDs (such as gonorrhea) can be transmitted easily through unprotected oral sex, but the risk of transmitting other STDs (such as HIV and HPV) is lower. STD transmission risks for oral sex decrease when semen doesn't enter the mouth. Ass eating (*rimming*), another fantastically entertaining activity, carries a high risk of contracting gastrointestinal bugs (such as amoebic dysentery) and Hepatitis A. So, if you haven't had a Hep A shot, barriers are a must for ass eating. (Those sleeping with a partner long-term often develop some immunity to their partners' butthole bacteria; this isn't the case for Hep A.) Some STDs (such as HPV) can be transmitted by sharing sex toys, so it's safest to use condoms when sharing toys (that way you don't have to break to sterilize toys). Plus, some sex toys are made of porous material and can't be sterilized, so condoms are a must.

Special concerns for three

When it comes to sex with three, there are several health issues to consider. You'll be using fingers, tongues, and toys on more than one other person, so it's critical to make sure not to transfer fluids from one person to another unless you're all fluid bonded. Always switch condoms between partners. Use condoms on sex toys, so you don't have to stop to sterilize them. If you've had ungloved fingers in someone's pussy or ass, wash your hands thoroughly before touching a pussy or putting them near anyone's mouth. Beyond spreading STDs, assholes contain bacteria that can contaminate pussies and cause infections.

Human immunodeficiency virus (HIV)

- **How to know if you have it:** Get tested. It is possible to be asymptomatic for extended periods. With standard HIV testing, it can take three to six months from the last potential exposure for the test to be accurate.
- **How to get it:** Vaginal and anal intercourse carry the greatest risk; transmission through oral sex is less common.

- **Cure:** Treatments have become much more effective lately, but there is no cure.
- **What you can do about it:** Use condoms for vaginal and anal intercourse. The virus concentration is much lower in vaginal fluid than sperm, so women who have sex only with other women are at a lower risk. The risk of transmission is much lower for unprotected oral sex (both givers and receivers) than for unprotected intercourse. Lower the risk by only performing oral sex with a healthy mouth, and don't allow anyone to cum in your mouth. Transmission risk factors for receiving cunnilingus are very low. The safest way to go is to use barriers for oral sex.

Herpes

- **How to know if you have it:** Most people aren't aware they have it. Symptoms include sores in the genital area or on the mouth. Get tested.
- **How to get it:** What does genital herpes have to do with cold sores on your mouth? Is it contagious when there aren't any visible outbreaks? Herpes is highly contagious, and it's most contagious immediately before, during, and following an outbreak—that means just because you don't see any sores doesn't mean

you're in the clear. Herpes simplex 1 (HSV-1) mostly occurs on the mouth in the form of "cold sores," which theoretically can spread to the crotch through unprotected oral contact. HSV-1 isn't the most common cause of genital herpes. Herpes simplex 2 (HSV-2), the most common cause of genital herpes, is transmitted through vaginal, anal, or oral sex. Herpes can be transmitted from genitals to mouth or vice versa during unprotected oral sex; some consider the risk acceptably low when there isn't an outbreak, others don't. You also need to know that herpes is very common: the Centers for Disease Control and Prevention estimates that one in five adults nationwide are infected with genital herpes.

- **Cure:** Treatments can help suppress outbreaks, but there's no cure. Herpes is not life threatening.
- **What you can do about it:** Use latex barriers for oral, anal, and vaginal sex. During an outbreak, don't have intercourse, even with a condom, as herpes can spread through areas not covered by the condom.

Human papillomavirus (HPV)

- **How to know if you have it:** Since HPV rarely causes symptoms, most carriers don't know they have it. HPV is so common that gynecologists do not routinely test for it during annual pap smears. An abnormal reading on a pap smear can diagnose precancerous cells caused by HPV. Genital warts also indicate HPV infection. Ask your gynecologist for an HPV test.

- **How to get it:** There are more than thirty strains of HPV that can infect the genital area—some produce warts, some cause cervical cancers, and others may have no harmful effects. HPV is the most common STD in the country; at least 50 percent of sexually active adults will contract HPV at some point in their lives. HPV is transmitted through anal and vaginal intercourse and sharing sex toys. Oral sex has a very low risk of transmission.
- **Cure:** There is no cure yet. Problems caused by some strains of HPV (such as genital warts) can be treated.
- **What you can do about it:** Use condoms for intercourse and sex-toy play. A new vaccine that prevents several strains of HPV that cause most types of cervical cancer has just become available. Get it. (Note: The vaccine doesn't protect against every HPV strain, so it's still necessary to get routine pap smears.)

Chlamydia

- **How to know if you have it:** Seventy-five percent of men and half of women who have it show no symptoms. Symptoms may include lower abdominal pain, nausea, fever, and pain during intercourse. If untreated, chlamydia can cause sterility, pelvic inflammatory disease, and other physical maladies. Get tested.
- **How to get it:** It is most commonly transmitted through vaginal and anal intercourse, and very rarely through oral sex.
- **Cure:** Antibiotics.
- **What you can do about it:** Use a condom during intercourse.

Gonorrhea

- **How to know if you have it:** Most men have symptoms, while most women have no symptoms. Symptoms may include a discharge and painful urination. Gonorrhea can be contracted in the mouth or throat, causing a sore throat. Get tested.
- **How to get it:** This bacterial infection is transmitted through vaginal, anal, and oral sex. Infected semen entering the throat can transmit the infection to the person performing oral sex.
- **Cure:** Antibiotics.

- **What you can do about it:** Use barriers during intercourse and oral sex.

Bacterial vaginosis (BV)

- **How to know if you have it:** Symptoms include an unpleasant odor, itching, and unusual discharge. Get tested.
- **How to get it:** This relatively common infection caused by an imbalance in bacteria, BV seems to be a condition that isn't sexually transmitted. Having a new partner (or two) increases the chances of developing the condition, and it's more common among women with female partners because there's an increased risk from sharing sex toys and inserting fingers. Women can develop it even when they only have protected sex with condoms.
- **Cure:** Antibiotics.
- **What you can do about it:** Keep the kitty clean and dry after sex.

Hepatitis A, B, and C

- **How to know if you have it:** Symptoms may include vomiting, fever, nausea, abdominal pain, and fatigue. Get tested.
- **How to get it:** Hepatitis A spreads primarily through anal play (including ass licking and

intercourse) and by eating contaminated food. Hep B spreads mostly through vaginal and anal intercourse (rips and tears make transmission more likely because it's a blood-borne virus). Hep C is transmitted through blood-to-blood contact (i.e., sharing needles), and is not commonly spread through sexual contact.

- **Cure:** There is no cure. Hep A and hep B usually make you really sick, then go away after a few weeks. Hep C stays for the long run and can cause serious liver problems.
- **What you can do about it:** Get vaccinated for hep A and B. Use a barrier for rimming, oral sex, and intercourse. There's no vaccine for hep C.

Yeast infection

- **How to know if you have it:** Symptoms include an itching, burning crotch and a white, lumpy discharge.
- **How to get it:** Doctors say yeast infections aren't contagious. However, new sex partners and marathon threesome sex sessions can increase the chances of getting a yeast infection. Pussies have delicate pH balances and introducing new pussy juice or sperm can upset that balance.
- **Cure:** Yeast infections are treated with over-the-counter or prescription antifungal medications.

- **What you can do about it:** Keep your pussy clean and dry after sex. Yeast thrives on sugar, so if you're susceptible to yeast infections, don't play with sugary foods (i.e., chocolate sauces) on your kitty or use lubes with glycerin (it's a form of sugar). Be careful with scented massage oils or lotions—many of these contain ingredients that disrupt the pussy's pH balance. Use mild soaps (i.e., Dr. Bronner's). Do not douche. Eating yogurt, which contains good bacteria that wards off the harmful populations, or taking acidophilus supplements may help, too.

Urinary tract infection (UTI)/bladder infection

- **How to know if you have it:** Symptoms include a strong and frequent urge to pee and a burning sensation while peeing.
- **How to get it:** Some women are particularly susceptible to UTIs. Sleeping with new partners increases the risk. UTIs happen because women's urethras are short and bacteria can easily enter the urethral tube, causing an infection.
- **Cure:** Antibiotics.
- **What you can do about it:** Ask your sex partners to shower regularly. Urinate before and after sex. Drink cranberry juice. Wipe from front to back. Make sure that if you're involved in anal play, your partners know not to touch

your pussy after touching your asshole—this puts you at risk of bacteria entering your urethra and causing an infection.

FANCY ACCOUTERMENTS

Finger cots and latex gloves

Finger cots are nifty latex tubes designed for a finger. These little finger condoms are perfect for ass play; when you're done with ass play and want to touch pussy again, just rip it off and chuck it, without worrying about which finger you used on her bum. And a smooth, lubed finger cot or latex glove feels way better in the rump than a jagged fingernail.

Dental dams

If your personal safety standards include barriers for oral sex, use plastic wrap or Glyde dental dams for ass eating and box munching. Dental dams are latex rectangles perfect for eating ass and bush. Put a few drops of lube on her crotch, put the barrier in place and dine away. (www.Glydedams.com)

Condoms

Lubed versus unlubed? Unlubed condoms are most versatile because you can choose your own lube depending on the circumstances. Some lubed condoms use silicon lube, which clashes with silicon sex toys. And lubed condoms often contain nonoxynol-9, a chemical that was initially praised for its sperm-killing qualities, but has recently been found to cause vaginal tearing that allows diseases to travel into the bloodstream more easily. Although lambskin condoms block pregnancy, they're much less effective when it comes to preventing the spread of disease.

Lubes

Lubes serve an important safer-sex purpose: they protect pussies and assholes from rips and tears, which allow diseases to enter the bloodstream more easily. They're especially important for ass play, since assholes can't produce their own lube. Most sex stores offer sample packets for lube, so test them out and decide which ones work best for you.

- Oil-based lubes (i.e., Vaseline, baby oil, and lotions): work well for massage and foreplay. The downside: unhealthy for pussies.
- Water-based lubes with glycerin: (i.e., Astroglide): thin, slippery texture and longer lasting than nonglycerin water-based lube. The downside: can cause yeast infections.
- Water-based without glycerin: thin, slippery texture. The downside: dries out quickly and requires reapplication.

- Silicon-based lube: ultraslick and long lasting. The downside: incompatible with silicon-based toys and difficult for pussies to flush out.
- Lube for anal play: gel lubes work best for anal penetration because they're thicker and last longer.

Okay, you're armed with latex and facts, now check out the next chapter for the nitty-gritty on sex positions that'll shoot all three of you to cloud nine.

IMPLEMENTING A SAFER SEX PLAN

Step 1. Get a complete STD test (including HPV). Ask your current lover(s) to get tested. Share the results.

Step 2. Do your STD homework and decide which risks feel acceptable to you. If you're fluid bonded with a partner, make an agreement about safer-sex limits with third lovers. That way, when you land a threesome, you won't have to stop midkiss to argue about whether your boyfriend needs to wear a condom when he gets a blowjob from another guy. Iron it out in advance. Be specific. You should both have a clear idea of how much you're willing to do with a third without using protection. Is it okay to perform oral sex on a third without using protection? What about licking the third's ass without a barrier? Write a clear agreement regarding safer-sex practices and both sign it. If you're flying solo, write up an agreement to meet your safer-sex limits and sign it.

Step 3. Read up on STDs until you have a clear idea of the risks associated with various sexual behaviors.

Step 4. Prepare a safer-sex kit. If you don't have condoms or dental dams available in the heat of the moment, you're much less likely to use them and to stick to your own safer-sex limits. Pack a safer-sex kit to keep near your bed. Include an assortment of safer-sex goodies i.e., condoms, dental dams, lube.

A few helpful resources for getting your facts straight:

www.sexuality.org
CDC National STD Hotline: 1-800-227-8922
www.plannedparenthood.org
www.medhelp.org/forums/STD/wwwboard.html (an STD forum moderated by H. Hunter Handsfield, MD)

CHAPTER 7

THE JOY OF $(SEX)^3$: POSITIONS, TECHNIQUES, AND INSTRUCTIONAL DIAGRAMS JUST FOR THREE

> When two people have sex, it's kind of like a campfire. When 3 people have sex, it's a huge bonfire. The energy is exponentially greater.
>
> —Stephane Hemon, seduction guru

There's a good reason threesomes are a porn-industry staple: they're hot. Not just a "Wow, that was great," roll-over-and-smoke-a-cigarette hot, but the kind of sublime, mind-erasing hot that leaves you seriously stumped about the spelling of your first name. So, beware: three-way sex may render you jelly-kneed, naked on a rooftop at four AM, beaming a million-kilowatt smile, and entirely convinced of your ability to fly.

The morning after I lost my threesome virginity, I went on a museum tour with my mother-in-law. Buzzing with a rock-star attitude and a threesome-savvy swagger, I was certain that fellow museum patrons recognized my sexual superiority. My mind kept darting back, rewinding and replaying every three-way moment in slow motion. No matter how fascinating the painting, my brain was squarely trapped in the three-way gutter.

But, for a threesome to cause such ex post facto obsession, everyone has to get off and that can be a lot to juggle. When it comes to bedroom gymnastics, every combination of three yields a different set of possibilities. (If you've got two straight women in the mix, a three-way daisy chain isn't gonna fly. But, the crowd-pleasing "club sandwich" might do the trick.) To find out what works best for your trio: review these three-way positions from A to Z. Then conduct your own experiments. Below you'll find the nuts and bolts of three-way sex including techniques, positions, and advice for handling the conundrums brought on by these debaucherous gymnastics.

> Sex lies at the root of life, we can never learn reverence of life until we know how to understand sex.
>
> —Havelock Ellis, sexologist (1859–1939)

TURNING UP THE THREE-WAY PASSION

> The fact remains that whether sex is being discussed or ignored, repressed, or expressed, enjoyed or endured, it is the single most significant aspect of our lives.
>
> —Diana Richardson, *The Heart of Tantric Sex*

Be flexible

There are infinite possibilities for three-way sex. And the first time you have a threesome, it might turn out that there are too many arms and legs to juggle, or for one reason or another, the sex doesn't go swimmingly. Know that sex with three doesn't have to be mind melting every time. Three-way sex can be a simple quickie just to help you sleep better; or an unexpectedly tender and intimate connection; or a light, playful romp with strangers. Don't pressure it to be one way or another. Experiment, play, and remember that each experience will be unique.

Check in

Don't assume everyone is totally okay with what's going on. Before things get too heavy, take a moment to ask everyone if they're okay with what's going on. Keep checking in. When you start doing something new, check in again. Make eye contact when you're talking. That sounds like a no-brainer, but often people don't make eye contact when they're talking. If you're still unsure or unclear about something, keep asking until you understand. Make it clear to your three-way lovers that you want them to let you know if they feel uncomfortable (or need to stop) at any point, and that you will respect their limits. If you check in and everyone is in agreement, then you've done your part to stave off morning-after turmoil and mid-sex drama. Check-ins help keep everyone from doing something they'll regret and open the lines of communication. When everyone feels they've expressed themselves, everyone usually feels freer to relax and enjoy, which translates to steamier sex.

Be inclusive

Those used to duo fucking will need to modify their style in the sack. The secret to smashing three-way sex is including everyone. It's easier to swing an all-inclusive threesome with a bi-curious or bisexual in the mix, but threesomes with two straighties of the same sex can work fabulously, too. This type of three-way presents spectatorship opportunities. It can be exquisitely sexy to watch and perform for each other, as long as no one gets neglected. So, straight people can swing hot three-way sex, too—it's just a matter of keeping the affection flowing.

Here are a few tricks to keep everyone included: While two people are having duo sex, keep the third involved with kissing, holding hands, or inviting the third to lend a helping hand. Another way to keep a three-way connection going is to rotate eye contact. When two people are having sex and the third is helping or watching, ask the third to keep eye contact with one of the two having sex. (Keep "soft eyes" that allow others in, rather than staring or scrutinizing.) Tantra gurus say eye contact deepens intimacy. Even if it feels awkward at first, go for it.

That way, when two pair off to schtoop, the third will not only be getting courtside seats to a live sex show, but she'll also feel like part of the action. Pay attention: find a way to include anyone who's been sitting on the sidelines for too long. Make sure everyone gets what they need to feel loved and turned on—that doesn't mean you have to play host and take responsibility for everyone else's pleasure, but stay in tune with your three-way playmates. Everyone needs to take responsibility for their own turn-on and that's the best way to turn up the sizzle quotient, but many folks aren't used to asking for what they want in the bedroom so sometimes it takes some readjusting to create that atmosphere. One young woman explained, "When someone is fucking the hell out of my G-spot, it's hard for me to suck cock at the same time. And since my husband isn't into guys, when we have threesomes with other guys, sometimes I've had to ignore my husband for a second. If the guys don't want to touch each other, someone's going to be left out for a minute every now and then." Make sure the attention gets around to everyone.

Middle Hog Warning

Meat in the Sandwich (a.k.a. "Middle Hog")
A third who monopolizes the sexual attention. Middle hogs hoard the three-way sexual attention, without giving much back. They may reel you in and leave you feeling bitter about not getting what you wanted in bed.

Don't play the director

Trisexual women often complain that men can be too aggressive in directing girl-on-girl action. Men: if you're in a threesome with two women, don't assume they're dyking out to please you and that you're in charge of the show. Back off. Be sensitive to what the ladies want and join in politely, that way you're more likely to get invited back for an encore.

> If [men] intrude clumsily, the women may subtly or openly treat them like annoying interruptions. A clever man patiently calculates when and how to join; often the women will appreciatively grant him equal time or more.
>
> —Arno Karlen, threesome scholar

Ask Sally Threesome

Q: I've had a double penetration fantasy for ages, but when we try the missionary sandwich position, we all get too hot and sweaty to cum. What should we do?

A: Lots of women have double penetration fantasies. In reality, it can be tricky to navigate, especially in a position that gets everyone off. Review the three-way positions. Experiment. And, if you can't find one that's going to get you all off, double penetration makes fabulous foreplay!

KEEPING IT IN THE BALLS—TIPS FOR GETTING AND PROLONGING ERECTIONS

> I only take Viagra when I'm with more than one woman.
>
> —Jack Nicholson

One common threesome hurdle is guys getting too intimidated or enthused to make the most of it. Many guys have fantasized about threesomes for eons and they're super freaked out when they actually land in the scenario. Throw alcohol and drugs into the mix and, voilà: soft cock. Review these tips and if it does happen to you, don't crawl into a hole and dream of time traveling back to that moment, just try again.

First of all, know that it does happen—especially to three-way novices. Second, lay off on the intoxicants when a threesome scenario's developing. And, relax. If you've hooked up with two bisexual women, you can sit back and enjoy the show. Tell them you want to watch for a while. (That may get your blood pumping). Or, tell them you just want to cuddle and talk. (That relieves the pressure, and if the three-way snuggle gets you going, a high-kink scenario may unfold anyway.) Another option: focus on pleasing the women. Yes, there are plenty of ways to fuck that don't require a cock: whip out a dildo, use your fingers or tongue. If that gets your plumbing working, great; if not, they'll still consider you a dreamy lover.

Another classic threesome fear for guys: releasing the ponies before the race is over. Here are several tips for prolonging erections and being an all-around awesome three-way lover:

- **Relax.** When an orgasm builds, normally the impulse is to tense all of your muscles. Notice when this starts to happen and consciously relax all of the muscles in your body. Tantra practitioners say, this exercise can open the door to full-body hundred-day orgasms.
- **Climb the mountain slowly.** Tantric sex gurus say that if you know a lover likes a certain move, do it once, then try some other strokes.

Then, return to the favorite stroke a few times, then return to other moves, and slowly increase the frequency of her favorite moves until she reaches the mountain top. Once she's getting close, don't switch techniques.

- **Don't be orgasm-oriented.** Enjoy the process.
- **Practice flexing your pubococcygeus (pc) muscle (the muscle between your balls and anus).** Without using your hands, try to start and stop peeing three times each time you go to the bathroom.
- **Masturbate.** Practice jerking off to the point of coming, then back off, wait, then start again. Practice holding off as long as possible. Tips for holding off on ejaculation: press your perineum (the spot between your anus and balls) to stave off orgasm (find the right spot and press hard—this can help you experience pleasure without ejaculating). Relax all of your muscles (especially your buttocks and genital muscles).
- **During intercourse, stay deep and keep your strokes short.** And, stop moving so much.
- **Take a tantric sex workshop or read a tantric sex manual.**
- **If all else fails, think about baseball.**

VOCABULARY BUILDER

D.P.

Double-penetration

When one person is penetrated by two others (either oral and vaginal, oral and anal, or anal and vaginal).

GYMNASTICS FOR THREE: TWENTY-SIX THREE-WAY POSITIONS FROM A TO Z

Try these positions to find your trio's favorite routes to three-way simultaneous orgasms or a three-way quickie. Some positions work best with comfortable bisexuals or gay playmates, others work for three straights; and, most of these three-way moves work fabulously with alternate gender combinations. Roll up your sleeves and get started.

A. Altar boys

One chick lies face up at the edge of the bed. Two guys spread her open and feast. Now, that's devotion.

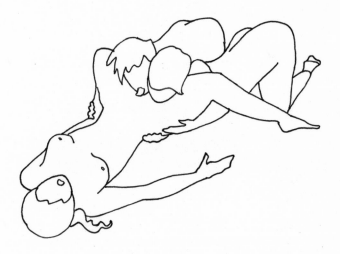

Three-Way Orgasm Rating: **

Best Combo: FM^2

Extra Credit: The truly pious will consider ass eating and fisting.

Difficulty Rating: Beginner

B. Backpacking

Two women bend over the edge of the bed, face down. The woman in the middle can spread her legs and lift herself on top of the other woman, so the guy can alternate schtooping one, then the other.

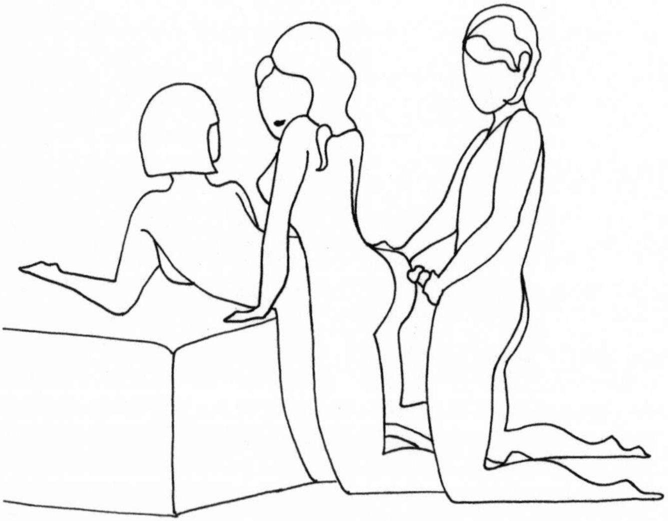

Three-Way Orgasm Rating: ***1/2

Best Combos: FM^2, $(B)F^2M$

Difficulty Rating: Intermediate

C. Club sandwich

A variation of the classic missionary position, the "club sandwich" offers the added bonus of an extra chick underneath. The woman underneath can grab the two on top, and press her clit against the woman on top's ass. Plus, the woman on the bottom can feel every move. The downside: possible death by crushing.

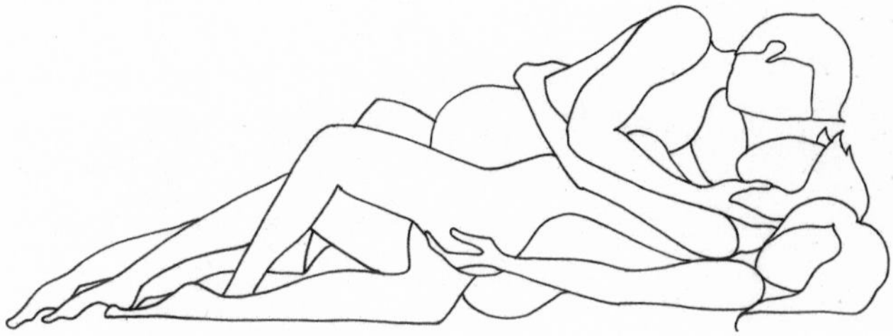

Three-Way Orgasm Rating: **1/2

Best Combo: F^2M

Difficulty Rating: Beginner

D. Double-penetration station

One guy lies on his back, while one woman lies face up on top of him. The second guy mounts the woman face down and slides his cock into her asshole. A D.P. dreamer's delight.

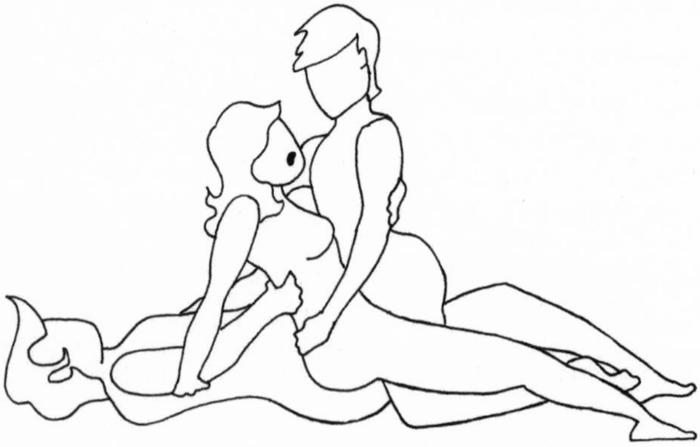

Three-Way Orgasm Rating: ***

Best Combo: FM^2

Substitution: Replace either guy with a woman wearing a strap-on.

Difficulty Rating: Black Diamond

E. Existential solution

One woman lies face up, while the guy kneels in front of her and schtoops her. The other woman sits on her face.

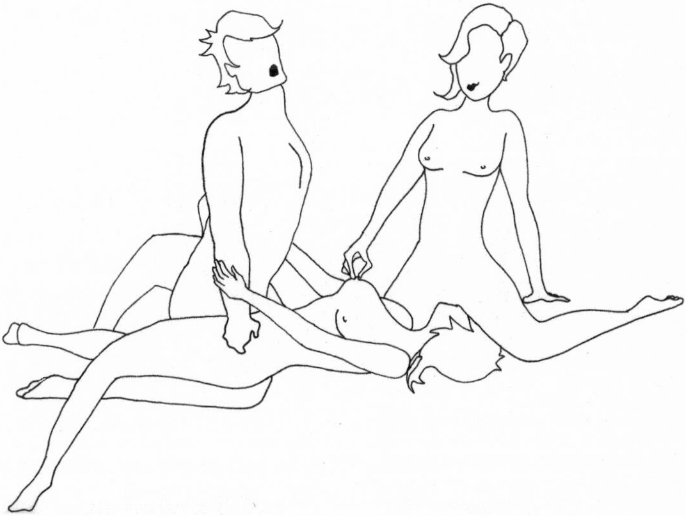

Three-Way Orgasm Rating: ****

Best Combo: (B)FFM

Extra Credit: The chick getting her pussy eaten can face forward and have her ass tickled by the guy.

Difficulty Rating: Intermediate

F. Feeding Frenzy

One guy sits upright. The woman sits on top, facing him, and rides him. They suck guy number two's cock together.

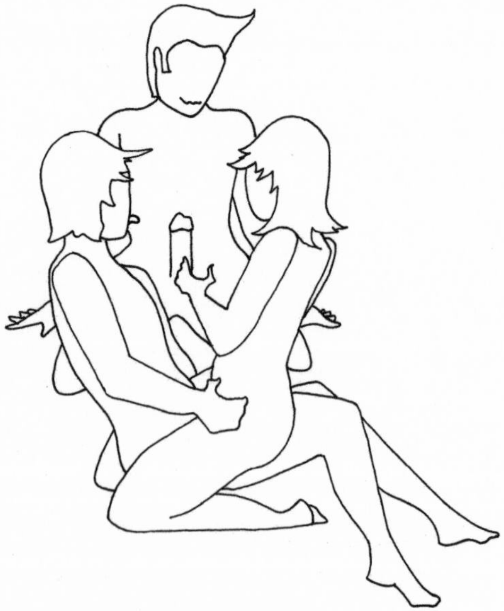

Three-Way Orgasm Rating: *1/2

Best Combo: F(B)M^2

Extra Credit: Deep throat to win.

Difficulty Rating: Intermediate

G. Greased lighting

Two women lie facing opposite directions; they spread their legs and grind pussies together. Clit-to-clit mashing can't be underestimated. The third watches and chokes the chicken.

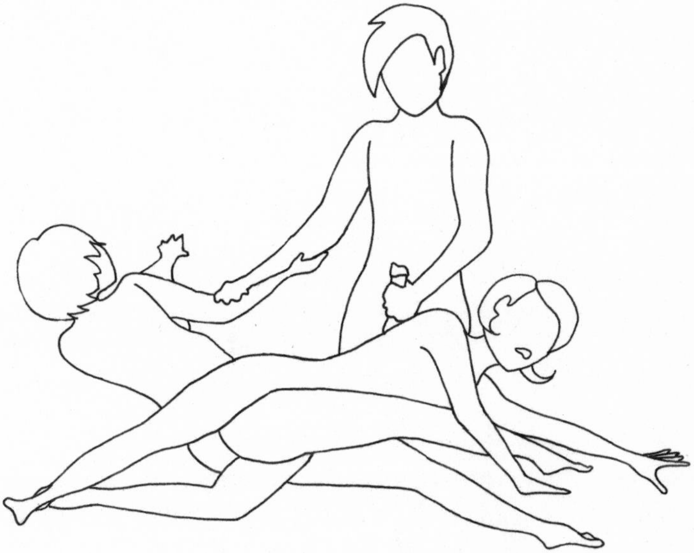

Three-way Orgasm Rating: ***

Best Combo: $(B)F^2M$

Extra credit: Fisting

Difficulty Rating: Intermediate (girl-on-girl experience a major plus)

H. Hats off

While riding a mechanical bull, she grabs one guy's cock and straddles guy number two.

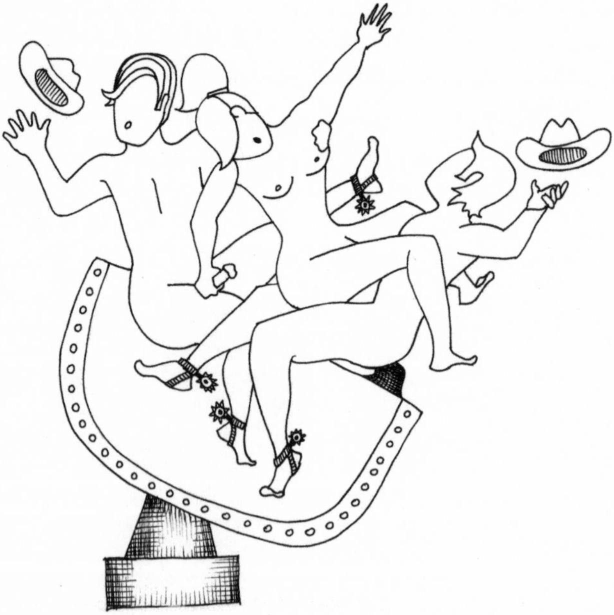

Three-Way Orgasm Rating: ******

Best Combos: FM^2 H (H) = mechanical bull or horse

Extra Credit: Add 1 lb. chopped celery.

Difficulty Rating: Double Black Diamond (circus and stunt performers only)

I. Icing on the cake

One woman sits at the edge of the bed. The other woman sits behind her. The guy stands off the edge of the bed and schtoops the woman at the edge. The woman sitting behind can grind her pussy into the other chick's ass and grab her tits.

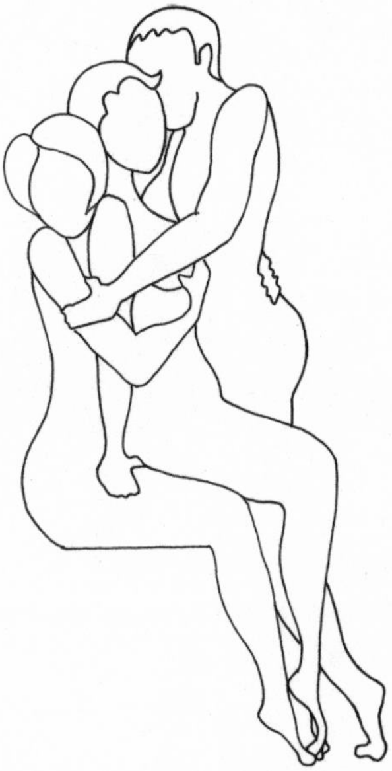

Three-Way Orgasm Rating: **

Best Combos: F^2M, (B)F^2M

Extra Credit: The woman behind can spread the other woman's pussy open.

Difficulty Rating: Beginner

J. Jousting

A double hummer yields triple pleasure.

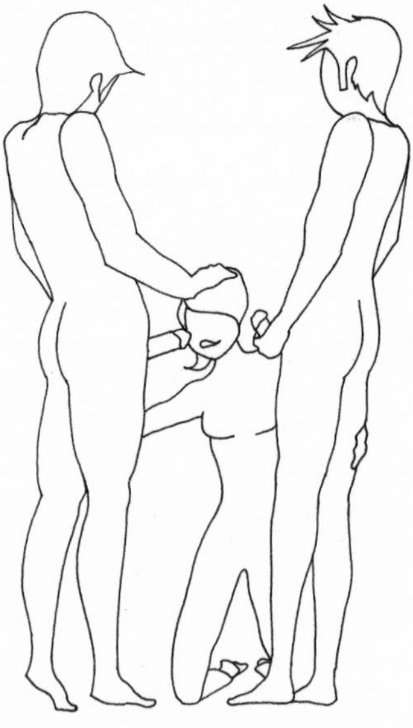

Three-Way Orgasm Rating: **

Best Combo: FM^2

Extra Credit: Clit play wouldn't hurt.

Difficulty Rating: Beginner

K. Kneading the turkey

The guy lies on the bottom, one woman mounts him and rides him cowgirl style. The other woman sits on his face. Facing each other, the women can play with each other's nipples and pussies.

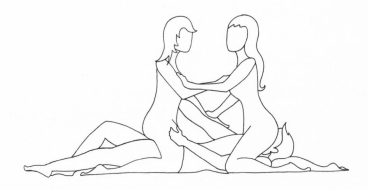

Three-Way Orgasm Rating: ***

Best Combo: F^2M

Difficult Rating: Beginner

L. Lower-case q

The black diamond of three-way sex positions, this one's bound to please those who can twist into the position. One woman lies on her back, while the other straddles her face (leaning up against the wall). The woman on top gets her pussy eaten, while getting schtooped by the guy. The guy can also finger the woman on the bottom. Getting the angles right here can be challenging, but accurate geometry translates to three-way nirvana.

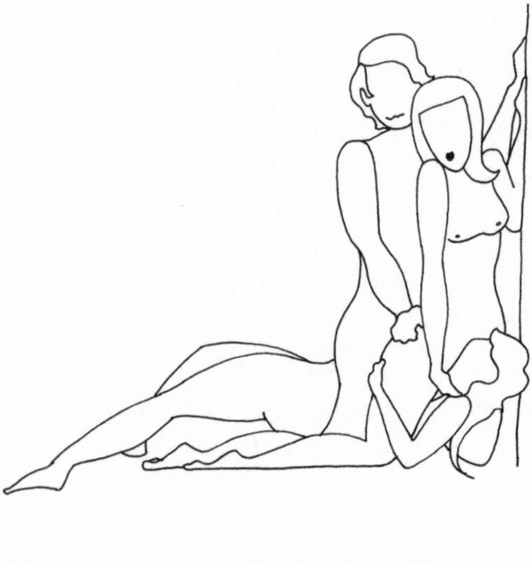

Three-Way Orgasm Rating: ***
Best Combo: (B)FFM
Difficulty Rating: Black Diamond

M. Mama's boys

One guy lies on his back, the woman lies face up on top of him. The guy on top straddles her face and she eats his banana.

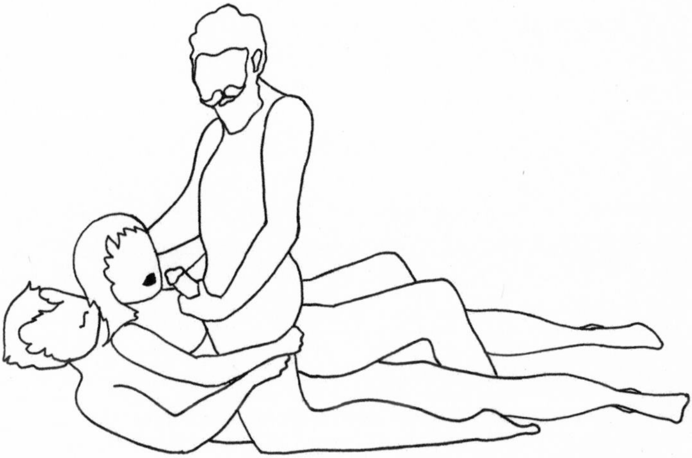

Three-Way Orgasm Rating: ***

Best Combo: FM^2

Extra Credit: She can play with the guy on top's asshole.

Difficulty Rating: Beginner

N. Nut crusher

An old three-way favorite, this classic position is a crowd-pleaser. The dude lies facing up, one woman lies on top of him facing up. The second woman lies face down on top of both. The two women grind each other's pussies, while the dude schtoops the woman in the middle. That's clit play and pussy penetration for the lucky lady in the middle. Getting into a rhythm here can be the trick.

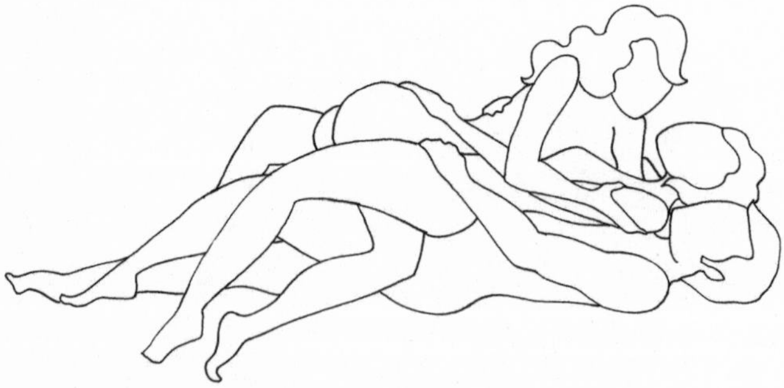

Three-Way Orgas Rating: ***

Best Combo: (B)F^2M

Extra credit: The chick in the middle can finger the chick on top's ass or pussy.

Difficulty Rating: Intermediate

O. Old-time carriage ride

The woman does a partial headstand, wrapping her legs around one guy's waist, while he holds her hips and fucks her. The third wriggles under to lick her kitty.

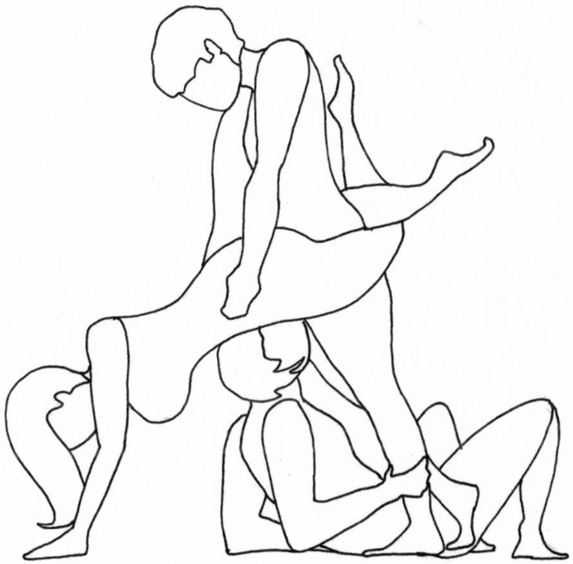

Three-Way Orgasm Rating: *1/2
Best Combos: FM^2, F^2M
Difficult Rating: Black Diamond

P. Puppy pile

The dude fucks one woman doggy style, while the other chick lies underneath and eats the top woman's pussy. The woman in the middle gets her clit licked and cock penetration at the same time.

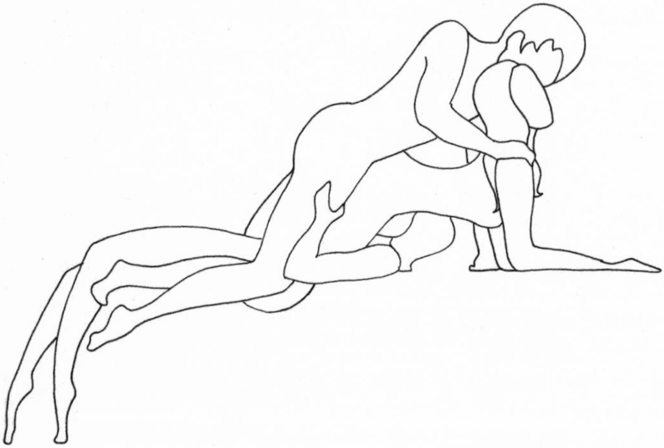

Three-Way Orgasm Rating: **
Best Combo: (B)FFM
Substitutions: The guy can be replaced with a woman wearing a strap-on. Another option: put a guy in the middle, so he's getting banged up the ass and getting his cock sucked at the same time.
Difficulty Rating: Intermediate

Q. Quilting bee

One woman sits in front of the other. The woman in the back fondles the other woman's pussy. Perfect for a peep show because the third can see everything.

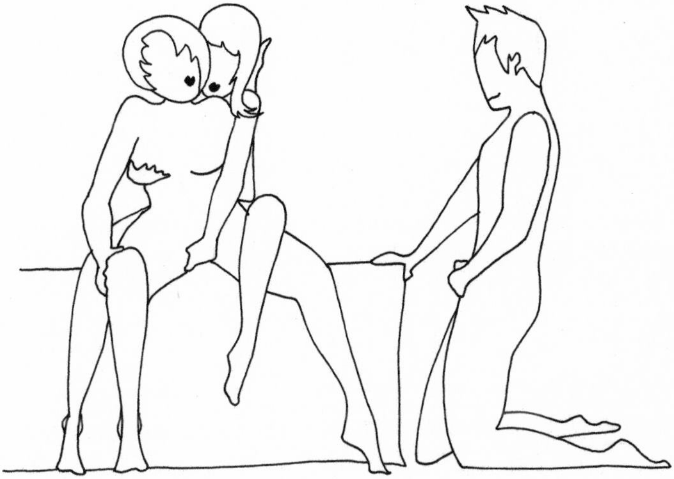

Three-Way Orgasm Rating: *1/2

Best Combo: $(B)F^2M$

Extra Credit: Tea for the ladies, please.

Difficult Rating: Beginner

R. Rotisserie

The top woman slides her mound on top of the other woman's pussy, then lowers her weight onto the woman on the bottom. They grind pussies together in missionary position. The woman on top can grab the other chick's ass to pull her closer. The guy schtoops the woman on top. To ensure even baking, flip the women before anyone pops.

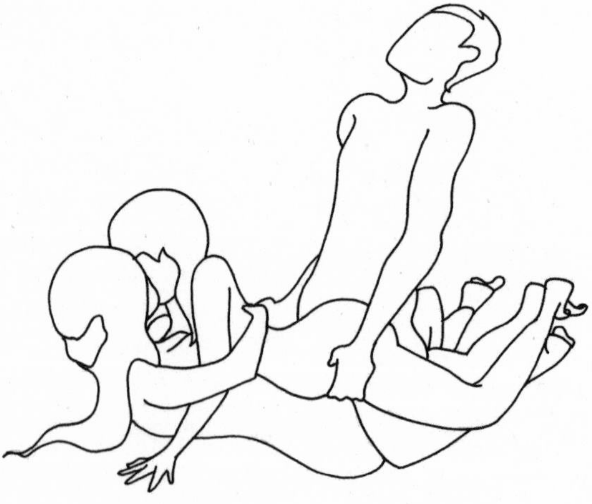

Three-Way Orgasm Rating: **

Best Combo: (B)F^{2}M

Extra Credit: Dazzle the ladies with G-spot stimulation and ass eating.

Difficult Rating: Intermediate

S. Seventy (69 + 1)

Two women munch each other's pussies, while the dude kneels behind and fucks the woman on top.

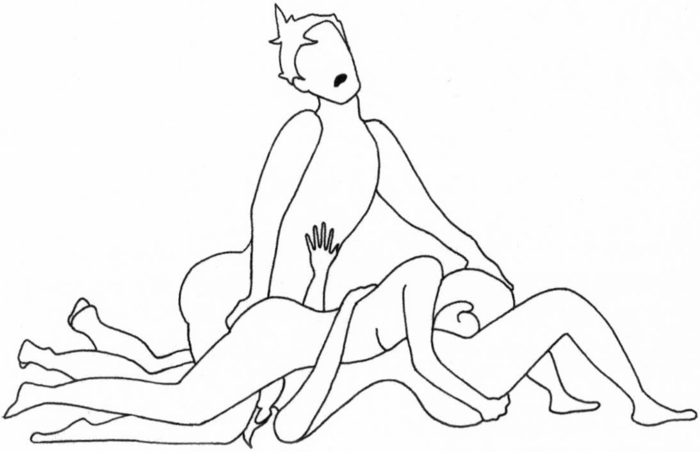

Three-Way Orgasm Rating: **1/2

Best Combo: (B)F^2M

Difficulty Rating: Intermediate

T. The smush and push deluxe

One woman lies on her back at the edge of the bed, the other woman lies on top of her. They grind their pussies together. The guy stands off the edge of the bed, and switches between fucking the woman on top and the woman on the bottom. (If all partners aren't fluid bonded, he'll have to switch condoms).

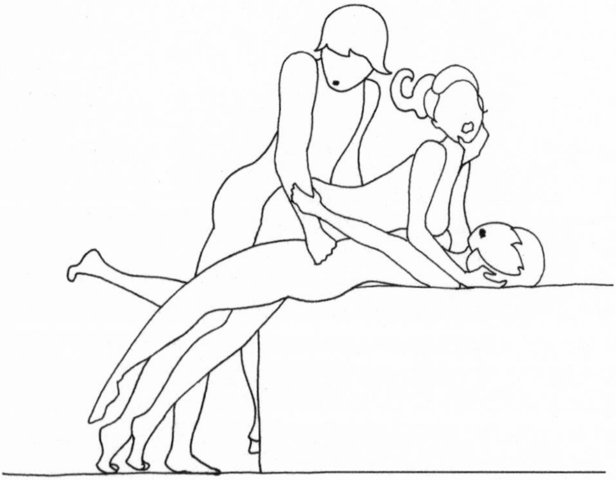

Three-Way Orgasm Rating: *****
Best Combo: (B)F^2M
Difficulty Rating: Intermediate

U. Upstanding citizens

One guy stands up against a wall. The woman wraps her legs around his waist and rides his cock. The second guy fucks her from behind. Another double-penetration special.

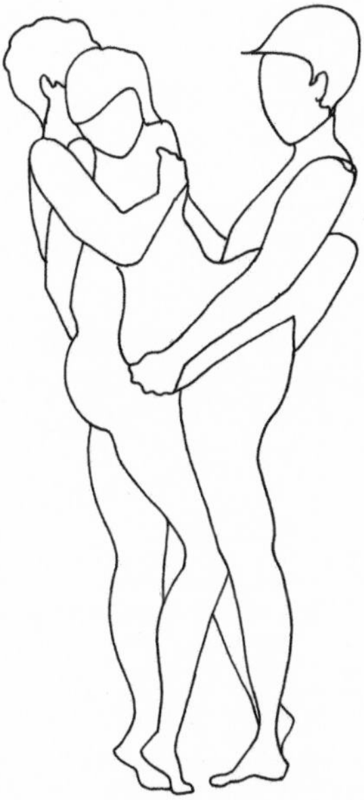

Three-Way Orgasm Rating: ***

Best Combos: FM^2

Difficult Rating: Black Diamond

V. Vice versa

The guy sits up, while one woman sits on top of him, facing him. The second woman sits behind him and grinds her pussy into his ass and grabs the other chick's ass and tits. A winner for trios with two straight chicks in the mix.

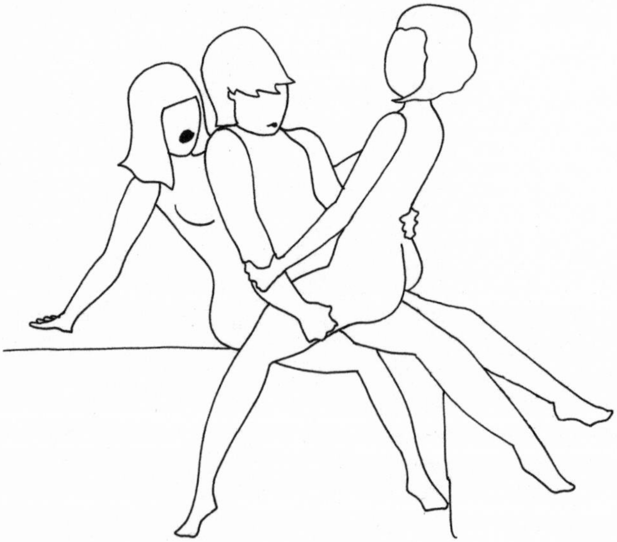

Three-Way Orgasm Rating: **
Best Combo: F^2M
Extra Credit: The women can suck face over the guy's shoulder.

W. Watchtower

The woman plays with herself, while watching two gentlemen 69 or fuck. And, if she's feeling frisky, she can cop a feel.

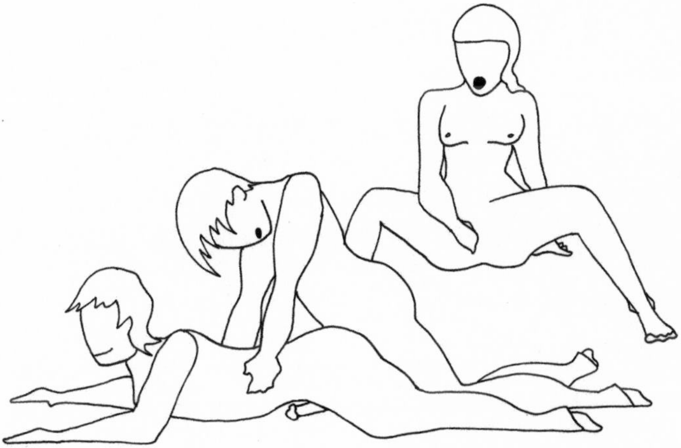

Three-Way Orgasm Rating: **1/2

Best Combo: F(B)M^2

Difficult Rating: Beginner

X. X-country skiing

One woman with a pole in each hand. What could be hotter?

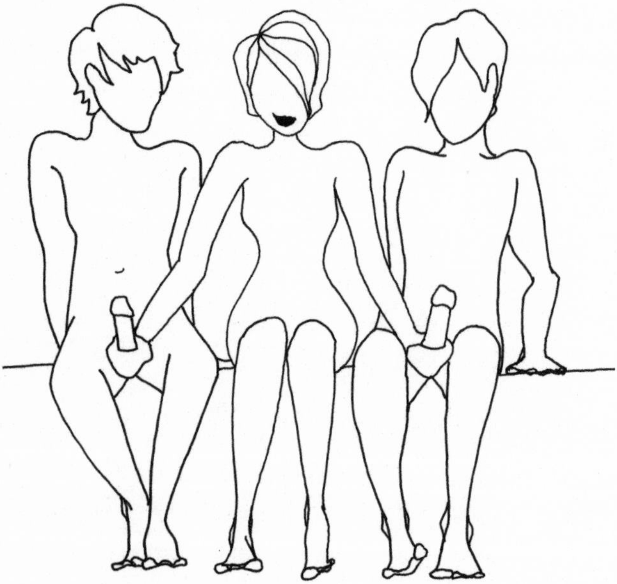

Three-Way Orgasm Rating: **1/2

Best Combo: FM^2

Extra Credit: A taste test wins bonus points.

Difficulty Rating: Beginner

Y. Young and the restless

One woman lies at the edge of the bed, while the other woman leans on the edge of the bed and eats her pussy. The dude stands up and schtoops the muffin muncher from behind. This one's a damned good quickie. The lady in the middle gets the double pleasure of eating pussy and getting schtooped at the same time.

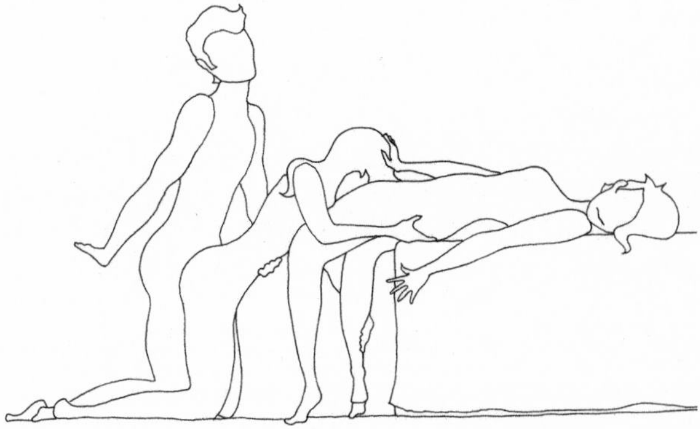

Three-Way Orgasm Rating: ****
Best Combos: (B)FFM, (G)FFM
Extra Credit: Mix it up with backdoor booty
Difficult Rating: Beginner

Z. Zen[3] *(a.k.a. three-way daisy chain)*

All three lie in a circle and lick each other's crotches. This classic three-way move works blissfully with the right combination of players. This won't fly with two straight chicks and a guy or two straight guys and a woman. With at least one bisexual or bicurious person in the group, it's a go.

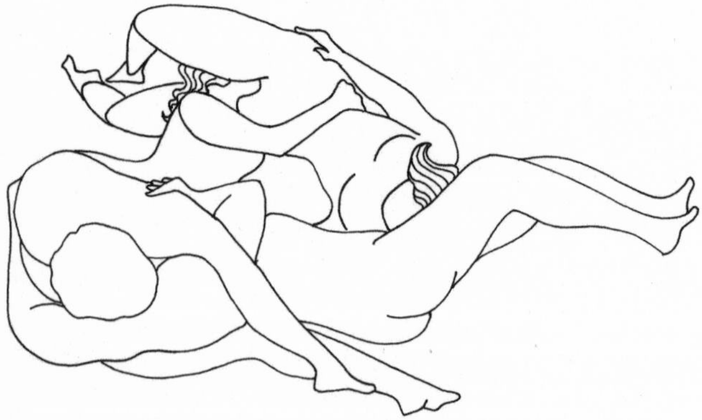

Three-Way Orgasm Rating: ****

Best Combo: (B)FFM, (B) MMF

Difficulty Rating: Beginner

True Tales from the Three-Way Pretzel

What I love best about threesomes is the way erotic sensations are multiplied. The extra hands, tongues, and breasts amplify the sensual experience.

—Connie, 41

I was surprised by how tender the threesome sex felt. There's nothing I loved more than holding my best friend's hand, while she had sex with my boyfriend. I felt so connected to both of them. It was really a beautiful experience that I wouldn't trade for anything.

—Zoe, 23

I find the position that suits me best. I lie atop Jennie. My arms are strong and can hold me up for long times so I do not crush her fragile frame. Sasha comes below and kisses her yoni. Jenn and I kiss. He penetrates her with his long, experienced fingers. His tongue and mouth caress her clitoris and it becomes engorged with blood and resembles a miniature penis. The Tantra master finds home and strokes her sacred space. Jennie begins to quake, shiver. She and I move as one. She orgasms again. And again. I merge with her. I feel what she feels. I feel what he feels. Our circuit is complete. We all feel what one another feels. For a moment in time, time freezes, and we go beyond time to timelessness. United, we three experience the miracle of love and divine grace as we look in God's eyes.

—Janet Kira Lessin, School of Tantra
founder and copresident
of the World Polyamory Association

My boyfriend and I had sex with a straight woman. I enjoyed pampering my husband and another woman for a while. I massaged her, then she and my boyfriend made out. I watched and masturbated. I got to watch the best live porno ever—it was fantastic!

—Jules, 24

I was at a party and I saw this sexy couple go into the bathroom. I assumed they went in there to do some blow, so I followed them. When we got in there, he said he wanted to fuck his girlfriend in the ass. I said, "Wow, cool." So, I licked her nipples, rubbed lube on her ass, and played with her clit, while he fucked her. She was so cute—she loved it. And, I can't even tell you how turned on I was by the time I went back into the party.

—Amy, 32

People often assume threesomes aren't as intimate as one-on-one sex. I've found that sharing a lover can be profoundly intimate. The threesomes I've had have been amazing experiences that allowed me to connect deeply to both partners and opened up doors of sensual possibilities unattainable in one-on-one encounters.

—Dennis, 37

I've always had this double-penetration fantasy, but when my boyfriend and I did it with another guy, we realized we all couldn't have orgasms that way. I was on top of the new guy and my boyfriend was fucking me from behind. It was doing a lot for me, but it wasn't working for the new guy. So, he masturbated, while I fucked my boyfriend. We had the hottest three-way simultaneous orgasm.

—Kathleen, 28

One night when I was a little drunk, my married friends started kissing me. She was really into me, but I'm straight so I wasn't into her. So, I ended up masturbating, while I videotaped them having sex. It was sexy.

—Liza, 31

TAKING IT TO THE NEXT LEVEL: STRAPPING IT ON, TOYS, ASS PLAY, AND BDSM

Ass-play basics

Wait until your lover is super aroused before experimenting with ass play. Start by gently pressing the pad of your finger up against his anus and tell him to move onto it when they're ready. Asses don't produce their own lube so it's key to grease them up so they don't get torn (gel lube works best). There's a range of toys you can use: anal plugs, strap-ons, anal beads, and more. If you're putting your finger up a guy's ass for the first time, be gentle and aim for the front wall, where the prostate sits—that way you'll hit the male G-spot and send him shaking. (Note: Be careful when switching from ass play to pussy play, use different fingers or use latex gloves. Touching pussy after ass play can lead to infections, so keep it clean). And remember: nothing says I love you like eating ass. Fans say it's the shortcut to bliss. So, flick, lick, and explore. It's safest to do this with a barrier (such as a Glyde dam or plastic wrap).

VOCABULARY BUILDER

Baiser

French verb meaning "to kiss"
(also, slang for "to fuck").

BDSM 101 (Bondage, discipline, domination/ submission, and sadomasochism)

BDSM activities range from light spankings to flesh-hook suspension and they're all the more fun with three. Think: Two leather-clad bitches tying a submissive to the bed. Clubs and events all over the country cater to BDSM-style kink; and the options vary from costumey latex clubs to hard-core private clubs (featuring "edge play," with needles, knives, and medical equipment). Many clubs feature orientations for beginners. Before you break out the whips, it's important to come up with safe words for "stop/get me the fuck out of here" and "slow down." It's also a good idea to state your limits clearly in advance. Then, experiment with clothespins (nifty nipple clamps), ropes, handcuffs, blindfolds, hot wax, ice, feathers, and other household items.

VOCABULARY BUILDER

Frottage

Dry humping. Pleasure sans penetration.

Dildos 101

Everyone prefers different dildo thicknesses and lengths, so don't expect one dildo to work for everyone in a three-some. And, if you're investing big bucks, find out exactly what each of your lovers want. Dildos come in an assortment of materials, shapes, colors, and sizes. They come in various shapes from butterflies to warthogs to AK47s. Materials vary: glass, silicon, or upscale "cyberskin," which sex-toy connoisseurs consider the Cadillac of dildos. Silicon dildos last for eons and are easily sterilized. The downside of silicon toys: they don't work with silicon-based lube and they feel like silicon. Glass toys last forever, they're easily cleaned and they work with all lube types. Rubber and "softskin" toys are made of porous material, which can't be cleaned easily (so it's best to use a condom if you're sharing). In terms of "lifelike feel," most sex-toy lovers opt for the "cyberskin" dildos (or a close cousin, VixSkin by Good Vibrations). Double-ended dildos are extra fun in a threesome with two (or three) women. There are hundreds of options on the market. The Vixen Nexus, a double-ended dildo, has great angles so it stays in place. Buying these products is much easier since many of the dodgy dark-alley sex supply shops have recently been replaced by shiny, modern venues exuding pervert-and-proud vibes. If you're still too squeamish to make an appearance, Good Vibrations offers a top-notch mail-order catalog and helpful, informed phone-sales reps.

Strapping it on is fun as hell

A strap-on is basically a harness and a dildo. If strap-on lovin' is an interest, it's worth investing in a decent quality harness, which can be pricey. Spend the bucks to get a strap-on that keeps your dildo stably in place (a wobbly dildo isn't sexy). Some harnesses come with fancy little pockets for tiny vibrators so the pusher can get extra pleasure. When purchasing a strap-on, make sure the dildo fits into the harness's hole—some harnesses have changeable rings to hold different sized dildos in place, others have a permanent dildo ring.

Okay, you have a fabulous harness and dildo, now what? Wielding a cock requires some coordination and practice so don't expect to be a virtuoso the first time around. You'll need to use muscles you've probably never used before and wiggle a bit to figure out the angles. (And you'll likely gain new respect for boys.) Doggy style is a good starter position because it's easier to get the right angle, to see what's going on, and to keep things in place. When it comes to strap-on sex, missionary position is relatively advanced. It requires balance, coordination, confidence, and knowledge of physics. When you're ready to try missionary, remember to watch your new appendage's angle and start slow. And it doesn't hurt to have someone with a live penis (or strap-on credentials) there to assist, advise, and point your new cock in the right direction. (Remember: if you're sharing dildos, use condoms so you can easily swap without having to break for a cleanup.) Once you've gotten the strap-on basics down, revisit the three-way sex position diagrams and test some new positions.

VOCABULARY BUILDER

Sexualwissenschafft

Literally translated as "sexual science," coined in the turn of the century, the term was used by German scholars to describe the new discipline of sex studies.

THE MORNING AFTER

Ideally, the morning after will involve berry pancakes, coffee, and a three-way quickie. If you've had fabulous threesome sex with someone who doesn't have their shit worked out on this (or if you don't have your shit worked out), there might be some humiliation or regret. So be a polite three-way lover by checking in with everyone afterward. Couples need to check in with each other. Ask: How did you feel about everything that happened? (Listen to the answers). Talk about it: What worked for you? What didn't work for you? Are you interested in hooking up with the same person again? Why or why not? Are there any limits you'd like to request in terms of future possibilities with this particular third person? What would you do differently? Learn. If you both agree, get back in the saddle. Since the third person doesn't have a lover to mull it over with, an upstanding couple will check in with the third afterward. Feeling like a couple's sex toy can be exhilarating in the moment, but some thirds may feel used or blue later. Couples: if you enjoyed yourselves, thank the third, tell him or her you had a good time, and ask if he or she is okay with everything. And, if you're all in the same social scene, it's smart to discuss boundaries and to talk clearly about whether threesome sex was a one-time thing or if you're open to future three-way encounters together. If the sex was sublime times three and you get butterflies when you think of your three-way, read on. . . .

THREE-WAY SEX EXERCISES

1. Competitive foreplay. One woman lies on her back. The two active players mirror each other as they give her a massage. The Objective: to explore as many parts of her body as possible, without touching her nipples, clit, or any orifice. Whoever touches an out-of-bounds body part first, loses.

2. Learning play sessions. A learning play session is an exploratory educational sensation session, which isn't meant to get anyone off. The idea is to learn which sensations each person likes. Many women think they can just think something hard enough to get their partners to do it to them. Instead of communicating what you like during hot sex sessions (which can feel dorky), request a learning session just for this kind of sex communication. Take turns with the active role. Play with different sensations: pinch nipples, scratch neck, etc. As you experiment with different touches, ask direct, specific questions: How does this feel? Do you like it when I touch you here? Or do you like it when I touch you like this? More pressure? Less pressure? That way, even uncommunicative lovers can express their sexual desires just by nodding or shaking their heads. It's less helpful to ask broad questions such as, "What do you want?" That dumps too much responsibility on the receiver.

3. A game to play: red light/green light. Touch one person in various places, when she says "green" she likes it, "red" means don't touch here, "yellow" means neutral. Take turns.

4. Complete a sex inventory. Complete the inventory yourself. Then, find out what your lovers want to try in bed, what they've already tried, and what they never want to try. Mark each activity: Done it, love it. Done it, would consider doing again. Done it, hate it. Want to try it. Might want to try. Never want to try.

Sex with the opposite sex
Sex with the same sex
Oral sex on same-sex partner, receptive

Oral sex on same-sex partner, active
Oral sex on opposite-sex partner, receptive
Oral sex on opposite-sex partner, active

Anal, receptive
Anal, active
SM, active
SM, passive
Vibrators and toys

5. **Bone up on your sex technique.** Take a tantric-sex workshop, a fisting class, or a sensual-massage lesson.

CHAPTER 8

RAINBOWS AND BUTTERFLIES, OH MY! WHEN A HOT THREE-WAY TURNS INTO LOVE

> Love is the flower of life, and blossoms unexpectedly and without law, and must be plucked where it is found, and enjoyed for the brief hour of its duration.
>
> —D. H. Lawrence

One night, my husband and I were at my best friend's apartment. After a few cosmopolitans and a game of truth or dare, we all ended up in bed together. And, the sex was so sensational that we started meeting for weekend trysts. One afternoon, I caught myself in a garden collecting wild butterflies for her. What the fuck? I realized I had fallen in love with my best friend. As it turned out: my husband had too. Suddenly it was a lot to juggle. He and I were still in love with each other. I loved them both, they loved each other, and they both loved me. The scenario was exhilarating and terrifying all at once. I tried to reconcile the picket-fence relationship I'd been living with this fucked up new three-sided mutation. When faced with the question of whether to follow this attraction into uncharted territory or to lock away the messy feelings for our next lives, I didn't know which way to go.

But, I discovered that loving and being loved by more than one person can be spectacular. Some of us have enough love to give two people . . . and, why not? There are so many cool people in the world and if you're lucky enough to meet more than one of them, is it really necessary to slam the door? One lover might spark your imagination, another might fire up your intellectual curiosity. There's so much to gain by experiencing deep connections with more than one person.

And just because it sounds off-the-wall and contemporary American culture happens to promote a different relationship blueprint doesn't mean committed threesome relationships are inherently not viable. In fact, people have been successfully creating healthy, long-term unconventional relationships for decades. Some threesomes stay together happily for decades (I even interviewed triads who've been together for more than twenty years). So, if that sounds appealing to you, there's no reason you shouldn't live the life you really want.

Committed threesome relationships present opportunities for living in a way that fulfills your craziest dreams. Beyond SEX^3 and an extra body to keep you warm at night, successful long-term threesomes enjoy a range of perks including another pair of hands to wash dishes, another shoulder to cry on, and another caretaker to sing children to sleep. Plus, there's an economy of scale, a built-in sense of community, a chance to open to love in a new way, and a release from an overdependency habit that kills many monogamous couples.

A threesome relationship might offer the support and love that fulfills your unique emotional and sexual needs, so go for it. (And who knows . . . you could wind up settling down in a long-term trio, moving to the 'burbs, raising babies together, and living happily ever after.) Even if a threesome relationship doesn't work for you in the long-run, diving into one could teach you to love bigger (with less jealousy and possessiveness) and help you discover more about yourself in six months than you could with a decade of therapy.

There is a tendency to want to put love in a tight frame, easily defined, and then put it on a shelf to over- or under-analyze. But love is far too clever to

> cooperate on this insignificant level. Love may park herself on a barstool and drink herself into denial. She may stumble aimlessly down a dead-end street, feeling lonely and sorry for herself, but you can't get rid of her that easy. . . . Love inspires us to be humble and generous and reminds us to leave our ego outside. Love begins, ends, begins, ends, starts off in the middle and then cuts you off at the pass. She flushes you down the sewage of loneliness and self-loathing, and then kicks your ass when you least expect it. Love is available when you're not, and sentenced to life imprisonment when you're on the prowl again. She just doesn't quit, and neither can you. See truly. Live fully. Think for yourself.
>
> —Wendy-O Matik,
> *Redefining Our Relationships*

So, just because love doesn't look the way you imagined, that doesn't mean you should kick it to the curb. The rewards of a long-term threesome can be mind-blowing, but it requires a strong commitment to honesty, self-awareness, and open communication. Without that, you've got zilch. If you're up for the challenge, talk to your lovers about how you feel. If they're on board, you'll need to custom design a relationship that meets each person's needs. Inside this chapter, you'll find pearls of wisdom on deciding whether to take a three-way sexcapade to the next level, advice on clarifying what kind of relationship you really want, an overview of different threesome relationship models, what to expect in a three-way relationship, secrets of a blissful triad relationship, and tips on living an unconventional lifestyle in the long run.

> Your task is not to seek for love, but merely to seek and find all the barriers within yourself that you have built against it.
>
> –Jalal ad-Din Rumi,
> Persian poet and mystic (1207)

THE PERKS OF HAPPILY AFTER FOR THREE

The rewards of a trio relationship can be enormous, but the readjustment requires learning lots of new skills, facing your own demons hard-core, and revamping your old belief systems. And the trip into greater self-awareness is one of the most intriguing aspects of trios. "There's a tremendous opportunity for personal growth in [ethical] nonmonogamy. It's the fast track. I think there's nothing even close to this except maybe a life-threatening illness," says relationship therapist Dr. Anapol.

The truth is: love ain't easy. And, love is even trickier to follow when it surfaces in unconventional ways. Serious relationships require work and when you're in one that your parents scowl at and mainstream society shuns, it's easier to quit when there's a bump along the way. Diving into a threesome relationship is like getting a PhD in love. Psychologist and author of *Polyamory: The New Love Without Limits*, Dr. Deborah Anapol says it takes a commitment to truth, personal growth, and communication to follow love:

> It's about being willing to let love lead, rather than your belief systems or your wounds. If you let love flow where it will, rather than trying to dictate where it should show up . . . if that's the kind of relationship you want, you have to find partners who can work that way and who are really committed to truth, both within themselves and with you.

> When you begin to touch your heart or let your heart be touched, you begin to discover that it's bottomless, that it doesn't have any resolution, that this heart is huge, vast and limitless. You begin to discover how much warmth and gentleness is there, as well as how much space.
>
> —Pema Chodron,
> *The Places That Scare You*

Intense threesome relationships can teach us to open to love in a much bigger way—with less jealousy and less possessiveness. Loving two also offers an ideal opportunity to let go of old relationship patterns, habits, and routines. Three-ways inhibit our autopilot programming and comfortable default patterns which may feel safe, but actually limit our possibilities for love. And threesomes can teach us to love ourselves at deep level. One woman put it this way: "When I first had threesomes, I always felt used. I simply couldn't believe that both lovers wanted me. I realized I felt that way because deep down, I didn't believe that I was really entirely lovable. When I really started to accept how lovable I am, I actually opened up to so much more love. It's incredible how much I learned about myself and love in general."

People in successful long-term triad relationships say once they've conquered jealousy and possessiveness, they ooze with happiness at the sight of their partner receiving love from another person. This overwhelming feeling is hard to explain to someone who's never experienced it. But it's true. Personally, I've felt inexplicably happy seeing my husband treated affectionately and adoringly by another. The love spills over and I get some, too. One woman who's been in several bliss-filled threesomes said, "A true threesome is about opening your heart and allowing yourself and the people you love to be the happiest they can be. Nothing does my heart greater joy, than seeing someone I love all giddy and in love with another wonderful person."

We all know people who keep "failing" in love; they keep dating different versions of the same incompatible partner and blaming their exes when the relationship withers. Then, mysteriously, the pattern repeats on someone new. These people never seem to see faults in themselves. But, while it's possible to ignore problematic sides of yourself in a twosome, when you've got two lovers telling you the same thing about yourself at the same time, it's harder to shrug it off. And personal issues that can be skirted in a twosome often have to be dealt with head-on in a three-way.

> Threesomes force you to see yourself clearly. . . . You have to be ready to understand that the world is your mirror. Your relationships show you something about yourself, so if you keep going through your relationships and blaming the other person, you're not going to see what you need to learn.
>
> —Stephane Hemon, seduction guru

Long-term threesome relationships can help dissolve calcified, unhealthy relationship patterns and radically upgrade duo relationships. Monogamous couples often depend on each other heavily for emotional support, family life, sexual affection, and social life. And relationship therapists say this overdependency spoils many otherwise happy couples. Bringing in another lover can defuse that unhealthy pattern. While threesomes won't fix couples on the rocks, they can make strong relationships even stronger by ferreting out deep-rooted patterns. And, singles shacking up with couples get the added perk of seeing the couple's relationship in action and, if they've got a healthy relationship, they can be fantastic role models.

> I feel like a lot of monogamous people expect their partners to provide everything—to fulfill all of their sexual and emotional needs. No one person can do that . . . both of my partners fill very different needs in my life. I've realized that one person will probably not be able to fill all of my needs and just because someone else if fulfilling them, that doesn't mean that it's bad or there's something wrong with my primary relationship. I feel that maybe I've chosen a better way.
>
> —Kristin, 38,
> who's been in several triad relationships

On a larger scale, threesome relationships present an opportunity for reinventing family. As nuclear families crumble at rapid rates and single career women in their late thirties choose to have children on their own, it's worth considering other options for creating families. And just because nuclear units have been the status quo in America doesn't mean it's the only (or best) way to be happy. In fact, many married career women today complain about the double burden (of careers and child rearing) that feminists in the 1960s decried. But there are other ways to live. In a speech to the National Organization for Women, lawyer and practicing polygamist Elizabeth Joseph declared polygamy the "ultimate feminist lifestyle" because there's an additional spouse to care for her children while she's out earning a living. Threesomes can shake up established gender roles by disrupting the default gender programming and requiring us to make conscious choices about how to divide household chores and childrearing responsibilities. Other cultures offer different, more communal lifestyles that allow children to grow up surrounded by lots of adults to shower them with affection—such as Israel's kibbutz system, extended family networks, or polygamous families. As more Americans experience a sense of loneliness in spite of living in crowded urban centers, it's worth considering other possibilities for reinventing love, family, and community. And threesomes could be just the ticket.

When a couple has an argument nowadays, they may think it's about money or power or sex or how to raise the kids or whatever. What they're really saying to each other, though without realizing it, is this: "You are not enough people!"

—Kurt Vonnegut, *A Man Without a Country*

Suddenly I realized—two people isn't enough. You need backup. If you're only two people, and someone drops off the edge, then you're on your own. Two isn't a large enough number. You need three at least.

—Marcus from the film *About A Boy*

We want to open our vision to accommodate monogamy as well as a plethora of other options—to plan for family and social structures that have growing room, that will continue to stretch and adapt, that we can fit to our needs into the future. We believe that new forms of families are evolving now, and will continue to evolve, not to supplant the nuclear family but to supplement it with an abundance of additional ideas about how you might

> choose to structure your family. We want to create a whole world of choices for sex and love, for family and community. We want to set you free to invent the society you want to live in.
>
> —Dossie Easton and Catherine Liszt, *The Ethical Slut*

> It is time to stop letting society convince you that you should feel bad or guilty about how many people you choose to love. . . . There is nothing stopping you from finding the courage to love as many people as possible and inviting them to help you raise a family, form friendships with your children, live in separate rooms, share lovers, share laundry, set boundaries, and start a minirevolution in the privacy of your own home.
>
> —Wendy-O Matik, *Redefining Our Relationships*

CUSTOM DESIGNING A RELATIONSHIP FOR THREE

One of the great things about threesome relationships is there aren't any prefabricated rules. There's no default setting, which means we get to figure everything out for ourselves and custom design a relationship that works best for every individual involved. The heart of developing a working relationship is finding a way to strike a balance between freedom and safety. What made your happiest

Up Your Clarity: Are You Open to Having a Committed Trio Relationship?

1. How much time and energy do you have for relationships? (If you're working eighty hours a week and raising five kids, it might not be the right time to start exploring multiple romantic relationships.)
2. How committed to personal growth are you?
3. How entrenched are your belief systems?
4. If you're in a couple, how solid is your existing relationship?
5. How comfortable are you living a lifestyle that mainstream society doesn't validate?

relationships so great? Consider what you need to feel loved and secure. Remember: everyone might want something different. Be honest about your own needs. Discuss. Experiment. Be curious about what the experience brings up in you; be willing to look and investigate. Here are a few models that have worked for others:[9]

A primary couple dating a third

This model involves a couple in an emotional and sexual threesome relationship with another person, who is "secondary." In other words, everyone knows and agrees that the primary couple's relationship takes priority and if conflict boils, the third will leave the scene. The downside: relationships aren't so easy to catalog, predict, or control and sometimes the relationship with the third grows more intense, or the third lover might want equal status. The couple should be considerate of the third's needs and totally honest about their intentions. The third person may be allowed to have outside relationships simultaneously. It's essential that everyone involved is up front about where things stand or else the third might falsely assume equal status. However, if the couple and the third are all open to creating an equal three-way bond down the road, it's possible to agree to this primary/secondary model with the option to change it into an equal three-way bond in the future. One soft-spoken twenty-seven-year-old brunette who's been married for six years and has had numerous triad relationships said, "I just don't have the capacity for too many deep, emotionally intense relationships. So the triads that make me happiest involve one intense relationship and one more casual partner."

> In imagination, threesomes might seem like hedonistic leaps into sexual freedom. In reality, the more people involved in a relationship, the more needs and feelings must be accommodated. Each person relates to two others individually and together—a nine-sided cluster of relationships. A threesome often requires not abandon, but the timing and tact of ballet.
>
> —Arno Karlen, threesome scholar

VOCABULARY BUILDERS

Triad

A threesome relationship

Trouple

A couple plus one

Usage: "Susan, Linda, and John are such a great trouple."

Primary relationship

A close, committed relationship in which the people are intimately involved in each other's daily lives—often financially, emotionally, and sexually. This relationship may take priority over short-term or sex-based "secondary relationships."

Secondary relationship

A close relationship which takes less time, energy, and priority than a primary relationship. The relationship has fewer shared values, commitments, plans, or legal ties; however, the relationship may include a mutual desire for a long-term connection.

Casual friends with benefits

Ideal for those not looking for a committed relationship, this model allows three friends to enjoy each other for friendship and occasional sexual pleasure. These "secondary" relationships don't involve too many daily entanglements such as sharing a house, finances, legal contracts, or long-term plans. The perks: plenty of three-way sex, affection, and companionship, without the limitations and obligations of a primary relationship. This model works well for people busy with art, childrearing, work, and anyone else who considers relationships a low priority. These arrangements can continue for years. The downside: they may lack depth and intimacy and are less likely to push you to grow as much or as quickly.

The wide-open threesome

This model involves more intensity than the "friends with benefits" scenario, but focuses on individual freedom. Everyone might live independently and all are free to have sexual relationships with anyone they choose. The difficulty with this model is that it can keep people on the edge of their seats; it's less predictable, it doesn't feel very secure, and it takes more time/effort for talking through challenges. These can last happily for ages, if everyone involved has the communication skills down pat. The upside: it's the ultimate freedom model.

The closed, equal triad

A closed circle of three, in which no partners are allowed to have extracurricular sexual relationships. The triad may choose to live together or independently. In this formation, all partners are considered equal and no relationship is privileged over another. This takes time to develop because most triads start with a couple plus a single. The difficulty with this model is that it might feel possessive, which is one reason many people become disenchanted with monogamy and consider a long-term threesome in the first place. Some committed triads marry, though the unions are not recognized by the U.S. government. Some threesome circles raise children together and remain together happily for decades.

> Most people place a wall around their hearts to protect them, sometimes that wall is a little too thick. I don't want to play those games. In our threesomes, we don't want a friendship with benefits, we want one heart. We want everyone to be equally in love with each other. That requires being open and brave.
>
> —Stephane Hemon, seduction guru

LET THE LOVE FLOW: THE SECRETS OF A HAPPY TRIO

As with any relationship, triads move through different stages, which could be labeled forming, storming, and norming. During the initial forming stage, everything looks shiny and you may feel super enthusiastic. During the storming phase, arguments start and questions arise (such as: how the fuck did we ever expect this to work?). During this phase, one might contemplate moving to a monastery or voluntary castration. But, with solid communication skills, it's possible to get through the storming phase into a norming phase, where the trio settles into a happy, healthy relationship that may not look like the Cleavers, but might be a hell of a lot more satisfying. The storming phase can require a heavy investment of energy, skill-set development, and talking time. Once you get that down, you'll hit much smoother sailing.

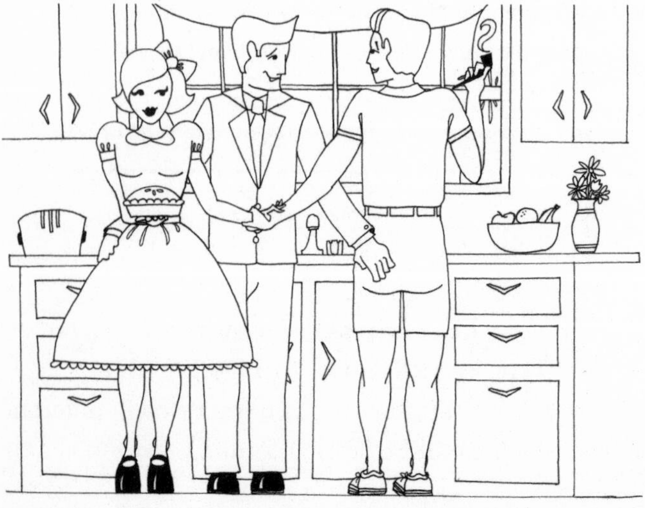

During the initial stage, new lovers often experience what polyamorists call *new relationship energy* (NRE), similar to what the rest of the world calls falling in love. With intoxicating endorphins surging through your bloodstream, you're apt to think about your new lovers constantly or tattoo three hearts on your shoulder. When NRE is flowing, you may feel invincible and suddenly quitting your job to follow Nomadic seafaring gypsies off the coast of Malaysia may sound like a brilliant plan.

> NRE has no relation to love—it can fuel it, assist it, hinder it, or prevent it. And NRE is at best a poor indicator of relationship success. . . . NRE is capable of overriding every grain of common sense. NRE is that wonderful and dangerous combination of lust and fascination that turns major portion of the brain off. . . . A real relationship doesn't properly begin until the NRE burns away. That's when you have to start dealing with this person as an all-around human being, replete with irritating little habits. When disillusion sets in, love can begin.
>
> —Anthony Ravenscroft, *Polyamory: A Roadmap for the Clueless and Hopeful*

These love chemicals are exponentially more powerful in a new trio relationship, which can present challenges for the established couple. It's natural for new relationships to come with a dizzying boost of NRE. When everything gets thrown into the NRE, both members of the couple might start to feel like their original relationship has evaporated. Plus, since it's most likely that each member of the couple will develop a relationship with the new third at a different pace, one might be more smitten at first and it's common for the other member of the couple to feel a bit bummed or left out. The solution: acknowledge that you're getting an NRE boost around your new flame, don't flip out about it, be aware that NRE is making you dizzy and don't get so swept away that you forget to give the preexisting relationship food and water. Nourish the old relationship too by spending time alone as a couple (sans your new addition).

When the NRE inevitably starts to dwindle, the trio dynamic shifts toward the *old relationship energy* (ORE) shared by the preexisting couple. That's when the new person is likely to feel insecure or left out. ORE means the couple shares memories and knowledge about each other. Founder of the Human Potential Center Bob McGarey describes the impact of ORE on the new person in the triad:

> They can talk about the time they went to Paris and the new person can't. . . . To make it work, it's

> important for the couple to be cognizant of the old relationship energy that they're leaving the new person out of and take steps to reassure the new person.

The solution: talk about it and offer reassurance to the new partner and build new memories as a trio. Watch the love, let it flow, and make sure it gets around to everyone. ORE and NRE are tricky dynamics to navigate. It's easy to get caught up feeling guilty about having such strong feelings for the new person and not wanting to hurt your preexisting partner's feelings. Then, as ORE kicks in, it's easy to feel guilty that the new person isn't fully integrated into the existing couple and worrying that the new person might feel left out. Don't fall into the trap of trying to smooth every ruffled feather. Instead, practice honesty and allow everyone to handle their own emotions. People in triads who know how to honestly put everything on the table make it work. Hiding how much you dig the new person isn't helpful and hiding how much you love your preexisting partner won't help, either.

The secret to managing the shifting energies between three is to stay clear on your own needs. If anyone starts kowtowing to the other two, everyone's likely to wind up with hurt feelings. That isn't a license to be an inconsiderate bastard when it comes to other people's feelings, but it's imperative to be clear and to express what you want directly. Telling mini-lies to make your lovers feel better or to stave off jealousy doesn't work in a threesome

Allow for the ebb and flow

Threesomes basically involve four different relationships—three relationships between each pair plus the relationship between all three together. Each relationship will evolve differently—at its own unique pace, emotional intensity, and sexual attraction level. It's impossible for both members of couple to develop a relationship at the same rate with a new person, so one member will likely fall behind for a while. This shouldn't be cause for alarm, just be aware and talk about it. Those shifting dynamics are natural. And as long as everyone in the trio has a romantic relationship with at least one person in the group (and a friendship with the other person), the trio can still work fabulously for everyone. Alternative relationship therapist Kathy Labriola says it's important for trio lovers to realize that there will be lots of ups and downs at first. According to Labriola:

> It's rare for all three to be equally enamored—both sexually and romantically at the same time. At one point or another, one relationship will be very hot and the other a little blah (in terms of sex or time and attention). And, it's important not to get totally freaked out by that. I have to reassure them that

> there are cycles to this, there are always going to be unequal levels of attention and interest. . . . I try to alert people that these cycles are just natural and normal.

To foster growth in the trio as a whole, each pair needs space and privacy to develop and deepen their relationship. So, plan special twosome dates for each pair (even though that sounds so twentieth century) and plan dates for the trio as a whole. It also helps to create a schedule that allows each pair to sleep together independently.

Vees can be sublime, too

Maybe your trio started as a hot three-way, you all had fabulous sex and spent hours lounging around eating Chinese food together. Then, maybe there was a twist. Maybe one relationship disintegrated (or never materialized) while the other two relationships grew stronger. Welcome to the "vee" triad. A vee is when one person has intimate relationships with two people, who aren't intimately involved with each other. If a triad evolves into a vee, don't assume it's spiraling toward a deadly love triangle and the whole relationship is a bust. As long as each person in the triad keeps at least one romantic relationship, vees can be sublime for everyone involved. Relationship therapist Labriola says, "It's okay if all three relationships don't flower into the most fabulous relationships ever. Even if it doesn't turn out exactly the way they originally thought it would, it can still be great. They're still going to be happy living together as a group in a triad, it'll just be a different configuration."

Vees take various shapes. A triad may be sexually a vee (i.e., two straight guys and a gal), or a triad may be sexually a vee but emotionally an equal triad, or emotionally a vee but sexually an equal triad. Or a threesome may have started out with two bicurious members, but then they end up feeling more like friends than lovers, but they're both still feeling attracted to the third.

Vees can also start when one member of a couple falls for someone new and the other member of the couple doesn't feel romantically attracted to them. Instead of assuming that the primary couple needs to end, a fulfilling vee might be an option.

Singles: the magic and challenge of joining a duo

At first, when the love chemicals are abundant, the new partner will probably have an easier time feeling included by the couple. But, when that initial buzz wears off, the new partner might feel left out or begin to question whether they'll ever be fully incorporated as an equal into the preexisting relationship.

So, know what you're looking for in the trio relationship. Reflect on whether you're looking for a long-term commitment with the couple or more of a friends-with-benefits type of arrangement. Consider whether you want to be an equal partner or if secondary status will do. Decide if you'd like to keep dating on the side. Once you've clarified your own vision, discuss your intentions honestly with your lovers. Find out their intentions: are they genuinely open to creating an equal three-way bond with you or do they want to keep the couple relationship the priority? It's important that everyone talk openly about expectations.

If everyone's on the same page and you decide to move forward, know that it will take time to feel safe and secure with the couple. Being the new person can be scary, so it's okay to protect yourself by moving slowly and cautiously. Don't feel pressured into committing too quickly or more intensely than you're ready for. Take your time. Don't make major changes in your life until you feel confident that the threesome relationship is really stable, intimate, and healthy. Especially if you're in a long-distance trio with a couple, don't feel rushed to give up your own life to move in with the couple.

Watch for (and unplug) power play

Most triads don't form from three singles; they usually form from a couple plus one. And herein lies the rub. Established couples tend to see themselves as a single unit, a voting bloc, with more power than the newly attached partner's vote. Even couples that try their best to be egalitarian still have a history and are more likely to vote as a bloc. That means the new person in the triad might feel expendable. That's a tough pill to swallow. When it comes down to it, if the triad isn't working, often the couple will eliminate the third. As the new person, it takes a strong sense of self-worth to feel safe and loved as the third. When these power dynamics surface, call them out. Talk about it. These power dynamics can be overcome with awareness, radically honest communication, and a three-way effort to equally share power. If the trio intends to remain a primary couple with a secondary playmate, then sharing power isn't part of the plan.

VOCABULARY BUILDER

Compersion

Happiness when your lover falls in love or gets a killer blowjob from another person.

Zen and the art of threesomes

Don't brush shit under the rug. You might be able to get away with your passive-aggressive habits and other bad communication habits in a couple, but it's impossible with three. Commit to practicing radical honesty. If you're upset or you're not getting what you need from your lovers, face it right away. Be willing to look at yourself—ugly warts and all. Learn to know what's going on inside you, so you can express it to your lovers quickly and efficiently. Be brave enough to explore any uncomfortable emotions that surface. Learn to ask for what you need clearly and directly (without pouting or shouting). Hone your skills. Commit to take your personal growth seriously. Read up on jealousy management. Take communication workshops. Meditate. Become a communication and self-awareness black belt. Know that you can create kick-ass unorthodox relationships. Practice this and your relationships will flower.

Build your allies

Relationships thrive in community. But your three-way might not be welcomed with open arms at your grandma's bridge club. So, instead of shouting your threesome dreams from the mountaintop and risking isolating yourself from your existing friends and family, start by finding other relationship adventurers. Reach out to alternative-relationship friendly coaches and polyamory/alternative lifestyle groups in your area; there are many diverse communities that support alternative relationships of all kinds, so check them out to find which ones work for you. Know that there are thousands of others around the world making freaky relationships work.

> Yet in time our threesome began to feel isolated, apart from our peers because we worshipped outside the church of coupledom. Hosts feel uncomfortable inviting a ménage to dinner and at restaurants there are no cozy tables for three.
>
> —Barbara Foster, *Three in Love*

And, if you've never been in an honest nonmonogamous relationship before, get help from the pros. There are lots of counselors, therapists, and coaches who know the ins and outs of alternative relationships. Use them. Delving into nontraditional relationships can feel like reinventing the wheel. It's helpful to find a professional who has experience with alternative relationships. These pros have effective tools to help you custom design a nontraditional relationship and to handle the challenges with grace. They can help you figure out if a triad relationship is right for you, decide what kind of relationship is right for you, and negotiate agreements and boundaries. Be careful not to use a mental health professional who pathologizes alternative relationship models—that cultural bias won't help (it wasn't long ago that psychotherapists routinely tried to "convert" gay clients). Once you learn the new skill set, you'll be able to create the relationships you want.

VOCABULARY BUILDER

Ménage à trois

Commonly used to mean threesome sex, the French phrase originally meant "household of three."

ORDERING A KING-SIZED BED FOR THREE

Just because most monogamous couples live together doesn't mean that's the best way to create a happy, long-term relationship. In fact, many couples crash and burn over roommate issues and plenty of stable, long-term trios live separately. So, let go of your preconceived notions about how relationships should be and explore the possibilities.

Negotiating autonomy versus group time is key to happily living together in any relationship and many relationships misfire from misaligned expectations about alone time and together time. So, before moving in together, consider your own needs and expectations about amount of personal freedom and privacy compared to family time. Are you all expected to be home for dinner every night or is it cool to go out for dinner with friends instead? Think honestly about your own needs, how much privacy you're willing to give up, and what you want out of living together as a triad.

Maybe you prefer to live alone because you want your own space or because your lovers are too sloppy. Consider other arrangements. If you can, share a triplex with three separate units, so you each get your own place. Or, in threesomes with a primary couple and a third or a vee, a part-time living arrangement might work well. If you all decide to live together, the ideal scenario would be to move into a new neutral space to eliminate territorial feelings and give everyone a fresh start with equal power, but if this isn't possible, try to make the space feel like home for everyone in the trio so no one tiptoes around like a long-term guest or a third wheel.

BREAKING UP AND MOVING ON: BACK TO MONOGAMY OR BACK ON THE MARKET?

If your threesome lasts till death, great, but if someone in the trio doesn't have a single love relationship left in the circle, someone's being chronically neglected, or someone finds they can't handle the social pressure of living an alternative relationship, a breakup might be in order.

Threesomes can be tough to break off, especially when the sex is phenomenal. Triads don't usually combust all at once and triad breakups carry unique challenges. Breakup pain is much easier if you are in a couple that lasts and when the dust settles—you've still got a boyfriend to drink martinis with—but, recovering from a trio breakup in a couple still has its challenges. If you're in a couple, indulging in breakup blues might leave your existing lover feeling like chopped liver. It's natural to be upset about losing a relationship, even if you still have one sweet lover to snuggle.

Solo trio-breakup survivors have a tougher spot for sure. The feeling of being abandoned by two people at once can be even more brutal than breaking up with one. The single might feel that the couple was more committed to each other than him. And, poof: there's bitterness.

And, the public relations problem of trio breakups compounds the pain. After monogamous breakups, friends offer lots of emotional support, but, after a trio breakup, they're less likely to dole out sympathy. Friends might take it as a delightful opportunity to rub salt in the wounds with comments like "What did you expect? Of course, it could never work!" (Notice no one ever says, "What did you expect? Monogamous couples are bound to breakup.") The lack of sympathy and validation after a trio breakup sucks, and trio breakup survivors who still have one lover are likely to get zero sympathy. Losing a relationship hurts. Period. Even when you've got another lover whom you adore.

Don't buy into the assumption that a breakup constitutes a relationship failure. Breakups can be constructive; they can salvage friendships and offer powerful learning opportunities. Even if individuals need to part ways at some point, maybe they enjoyed a successful connection for ten wonderful years or twenty-four amazing hours. There's no need to write off the entire relationship as a "failure" because it didn't last forever.

And, just because a first threesome doesn't work in the long run, that doesn't mean all triad relationships are doomed. One relationship breakup shouldn't be the death knell for creatively redefining your relationships, if that's your path. Chances are, you learned a lot from your first trio, and now you have a clearer idea about what works for you and what doesn't. If you've discovered that monogamy works best for you, then, good, you've learned something. And, hopefully, you've come out a better, stronger person. But, if the prospect of reinventing relationships still excites you, know that alternative relationships do work. And, get back on the horse.

COMING OUT OF THE CLOSET: ASSESSING THE PROS AND CONS

We all have secret selves. Such secrets want telling.

—Kenji Yoshino, law professor, Yale University

If you do decide to stray from the path of monogamous coupledom to radically revolutionize your relationships (whatever that means for you), you'll have to decide how open you're going to be about it. Everyone feels differently about whether to be open about their lifestyle or lovers. Couples indulging in occasional three-way romps often don't divulge this to coworkers, family members, or friends. Mom doesn't necessarily have to know you like to take it up the rump with a strap-on. However, when you're making decisions about who to love and how to create a family that makes you happy, you may not want to hide anymore. If your threesome relationship evolves in something longer term or if your marriage is open for the long term or if you decide you want to create a trio family, you've got to at least contemplate telling the truth to friends and family.

In the pre-Stonewall era, thousands of lesbian and gay couples lived in long-term relationships without outing themselves to friends and family. Today, many ethical nonmonogamists living in long-term threesomes, moresomes, and open relationships are still closeted. Many of those who have been living in triad relationships for decades still choose not to come out to friends and family. Some long-term triads (or quads) tell friends they live together for financial reasons. Other trio lovers enact don't-ask-don't-tell policies, rendering the trio an "open secret" of sorts, in which friends and relatives may suspect, without ever discussing the matter openly. That's a legitimate choice considering the possible consequences of coming out as nonmonogamous in America today.

It may seem strange, but "coming out" as openly nonmonogamous can result in more trouble than being exposed as a lying, cheating adulterer in a conventional relationship. Secret cheating (a treat that many marriages and long-term relationships enjoy) might be met with a slap on the wrist, while being open and proud about loving two (or more) people can jeopardize careers and even child custody. There are pros and cons to being open about your love choices. Being open about a stigmatized lifestyle isn't a cakewalk.

Sure, millions of suburban couples pass for the Cleavers, while secretly having little swinging flings on the side, but the truth is: secrecy sucks. You can probably convince your mom that you're sharing a bed with your two best friends because you can't afford heat, but that can be exhausting and stressful. And lying about relationships compounds the feeling that you're doing something shameful or wrong. Beyond the stress of lying to friends and family, if you end up in a longer-term triad relationship, your lover(s) might feel hurt if you keep them a secret. This can be especially true when a couple doesn't tell friends and family about extramarital lovers; this scenario may leave the third feeling like a scorned mistress.

> I grew up in a closed quad with two moms and two dads. They stayed together for twenty-five years. It was such an amazing, supportive, and loving family to grow up in. The only difficult thing was that we had to keep it a secret—that was the most challenging part.
>
> —Karen, 31

Do it for your country

Another good reason to be open about your love choices is to make the world a better place. Social change simply doesn't happen until someone is willing to take personal risks. Even the small action of openly being yourself can be revolutionary—it can create tiny ripples that eventually affect the way people think and live. The gay rights movement showed that coming out of the closet in large numbers can have sweeping social, legal, and political consequences. Although there's still a long way to go, gay and lesbian love has started inching toward mainstream acceptability largely because millions of Americans know openly gay neighbors, kids, and coworkers. That couldn't have happened without a massive migration out of the closet. But when it comes to trisexuals, polyamorous, kinksters, and moderns, there's much less incentive to come out because many of these pervs can easily pass as apple-pie monogamists. And the privileges of conforming are tempting. So, the growing numbers of ethical non-monogamists have largely chosen to stay in the closet; in fact, they're so hidden that many people don't even know ethical nonmonogamy exists.

Yale law professor Kenji Yoshino argues we are all pressured to "cover" or to downplay stigmatized traits to blend into the mainstream. We do this in various ways—by hiding hearing aids or changing ethnic-sounding names to commercially viable ones. It's time for a new era in civil rights, in which we are all encouraged to be open and truthful about how we don't conform to mainstream values.

> To be nobody but yourself in world that's doing its best to make you somebody else, is to fight the hardest battle you are ever going to fight.
>
> —e. e. cummings

Sharing the news: jaw-droppers, curious types, and fellow freaky lovers

If you decide to be open about your unconventional love interests, prepare for some raised eyebrows. Even if you're floating on air from your new three-way adventures, don't expect everyone to be as thrilled about your new trisexual zest. Some friends will think you're out of your mind. Others will exhibit zero curiosity and avoid you like the plague, fearing you might be trying to land them in the sack or convert their husbands or wives into nymphos. Couples who are ultra-secure in their relationships are likely to be curious and interested in having conversations about it; while those involved in secret affairs or who have unarticulated desires to pursue other lovers are more likely to be threatened when the topic comes up—and more likely to shun anyone who brings those issues up.

The news can be a shock; so don't expect your friends and family to immediately celebrate your three-way love. Be patient. Often, it takes some people time to digest and understand the information. Some who are initially adamantly opposed to the scenario may become supportive and perhaps even curious about how to swing their own unorthodox love interests. You might find that being open about your life allows others to do the same. Plus, you might receive some lascivious invitations from friends you never expected.

My experience coming out to friends as a three-way

pervert was fascinating, exhilarating, and at times, isolating. After several months in our trio relationship, my husband and I started telling friends about our girlfriend. Even some of our most "progressive" friends didn't take the news well. "The secret to a happy marriage is sharing a girlfriend?" Was generally followed by a searing silence. No one seemed to mind the concept of an occasional three-way fling with a stranger, but the concept of dating a third person was a bit much for polite company. Once we told a few friends, the news circulated at record speed via mysterious transcontinental gossip byways. Instead of seeing our new girlfriend as a trophy, many friends saw her as something akin to a disfiguring goiter—something clearly at the forefront of their minds, but far too distasteful to actually bring up. And most assumed our new girlfriend was evidence that our once-happy marriage had withered on the vine.

Considering the images of monogamous coupledom everywhere, most monogamists don't even know there are other options for happy relationships, so they're likely to be naysayers if you tell them about your love interests. Even well-meaning monogamists tend to dole out advice that can feed doubt and chip away at a potentially successful nontraditional relationship. No matter how many failed relationships they've suffered, those who lack experience with ethical nonmonogamy may see monogamy as the only healthy, viable relationship form. And, for those just starting to explore alternative relationships, that promonogamy cultural bias isn't exactly helpful. Don't let your pals' biases dampen your dreams.

Etiquette for Dealing with Square Friends

"Plus one" on wedding invitations and baby showers can be a bummer for trisexuals. In couple-obsessed America, you're unlikely to garner a third setting at the company holiday dinner unless you spin an elaborate fib or come out as a trisexual. Obviously, not all hosts will readily accept a three-way romance as legitimate; but, if you haven't told them, you haven't even given them the chance to gallantly accept your three-way flame. If the host still refuses to pony up the extra invitation, don't have a tantrum and refuse to attend the event. Emily Post wouldn't approve. Have a shred of kindness when dealing with more traditional friends.

> The future is not so much that monogamy becomes extinct but that it becomes one of many possibilities.
>
> —Deborah Anapol, PhD, *Polyamory: The New Love Without Limits*

BREAKING IT TO YOUR FRIENDS AND FAMILY

Advice for coming out about your trisexuality or unusual love interests:

- Establish a support system of other relationship adventurers first.
- Wait until your relationship is strong and stable enough to weather the challenges of coming out. Just like coming out as a gay couple twenty years ago, being open about unconventional love choices often generates some relationship stress and can destabilize a blooming relationship, so alternative relationship counselors recommend waiting until your relationship is healthy, stable, and strong enough to face the challenges of coming out.[10]
- Tell a friend or family member least likely to get their knickers in a knot over the issue, and, preferably, someone who won't blab to everyone about it.
- Test the waters first. Start by mentioning an article you read about open relationships or threesomes. If your friend shouts, "Those motherfuckers are going to hell!" reconsider outing yourself. If the friend shows interest or support, consider spilling the beans.

Let your freak flag fly

As more Americans live lonely, virtual existences—isolated in air-conditioned homes, communing through keyboards and plasma screens—it's our responsibility to seek out innovative ways to bring more joy and human contact into our lives. And it's worth looking at how mainstream images of love limit our options; it's worth challenging conventional prescriptions of how to live happily ever after; it's worth inviting more love into our lives; and it's worth experimenting with new ways to forge meaningful connections. We need to take risks to realize dreams that don't conform to the status quo.

From the standpoint of integrity, I think we all need to own up to our dirty little secrets. I believe that when we are open about our own strange desires or unusual lives, it paves the way for others to do the same. In the past thirty years, gay men and lesbians took a lot of flack to tell the truth about their love lives and their courage opened the door for a mass migration out of the closet. We're now at a moment in time when unconventional families (even thirty-year triads and gay couples) are losing their children in custody battles because their families don't conform to mainstream ideas about what a family should be. Given this context, I want to be someone who stands up for my choices even if they're unpopular, even if I get snickers at cocktail parties.

Now, this all sounds well and good on paper, but

when it comes down to actually going public with my own pervy ways, I'm slightly less certain. Do I really want my eighty-year-old Czech father reading about my three-way daisy chain? Even as I write this book, I'm standing on the edge, wondering whether to use my real name. There are consequences to consider: Do I really want my colleagues in academia to know? Do I want to be forever branded a deviant? Friends may assume I'm trying to lure them into my boudoir. Lecherous creeps may consider me an easy target. When I'm sixty, will I look back and cringe?

But, recently, I've begun to see my own slightly unusual romances as a welcome challenge in the world. I'm starting to feel like the price of coming out to friends (at least) has been worth it. It's been a culling process, in my mind. Those who can't handle it are welcome to ask questions and those deeply disturbed by it may have to move along. It certainly touches an uncomfortable nerve for many people. I've found that the topic elicits strong reactions one way or another—from prurient interest, to uptight bristling and pursed lips, to intense conversations about the nature of love.

Everyone knows threesomes are super-sexy, but they really fascinate me because they call us to question the received wisdom of our time. Threesomes can inspire us to dream big about the future and rethink how we choose to make our lives, how to invite deeper connections with others, and how to create new kinds of families. Three-ways also intrigue me because they offer uniquely powerful opportunities to chip away at our own protective layers and transcend the painful emotional debris that clogs our hearts.

Recently, friends and acquaintances have been coming out of the woodwork to tell me that they, too, have experimented with threesomes or open relationships and that they have secret dreams of reinventing their love lives. And some have been seeking encouragement or guidance on managing it all. That's an unexpected gift, and I'm happy to oblige.

www.threesomehandbook.com

APPENDIX A

COMMUNCATION ACTIVITIES AND RESOURCES

1. Exercise: Dream Scenario and Bottom-Line Scenario. This strategy works well for negotiating happy solutions between partners who don't agree. Try using this technique to discuss which relationship model appeals most to you. First, consider your ideal relationship scenario and your least favorite relationship scenario that you'd still be happy with. Then, sit down together and share your dream scenarios and your bottom-line scenarios. Consider where your visions overlap.

2. Exercise: Sharing Secrets. Time yourself. Spend twenty minutes taking turns with this exercise. You say,

"There's something I haven't told you." Your partner says, "Would you like to tell me?" You say, "Yes . . ." Then your partner says, "Thank you." The point of the exercise is to provide a safe place to express yourself, without receiving any comment from your partner. Anything brought up during this exercise should not be brought up later. If your partner drops a major bomb on you, you can say, "It's time to conclude the session today." Then, take a break. Although nothing interesting might come up the first few times you play this game, it's an awesome habit to get into, and deep fears and concerns start coming out later.

3. Exercise: Compassionate Communication. Here's a very boiled-down version of Marshall Rosenberg's compassionate communication technique—it works fabulously for discussing threesomes and just about anything. For example, after a threesome, try applying this technique to talk about it. Write your responses down independently, then share them with each other.

1. What worked for you about the threesome?
2. What didn't work for you?
3. What do you really want?
4. Then, make a specific, doable request.

4. Exercise: Active Listening 101. The first person talks, while the other listens. The second person recaps what the first said, then asks, "Is that correct?" The first person can clarify. The second person asks, "Is there more?" Each person talks for about ten minutes. Take turns. Rules: (1) Honesty. (2) After the talk session, topics raised should not be raised outside this setting. The promise: fears get raised in a safe container so they don't leak into other areas of life, and the others listen without jumping in to solve everything.

COMMUNICATION RESOURCES

Blanton, Brad, PhD. *Radical Honesty: How to Transform Your Life by Telling the Truth.* New York: Dell Publishing, 1994.

Rosenberg, Marshall, PhD. *Nonviolent Communication: A Language of Life: Create Your Life, Your Relationships, and Your World in Harmony with Your Values.* Encinitas, CA: Puddledancer Press, 2003.

Rosenberg, Marshall. *Being Me, Loving You: A Practical Guide to Extraordinary Relationships.* Encinitas, CA: Puddledancer Press, 2005.

McGarey, Bob. *The Poly Communication Survival Kit.* Austin, TX: The Human Potential Center. (Order online at www.humanpotentialcenter.org).

The Center for Nonviolent Communication—specializes in a unique communication technique that's super helpful for relationships. Check out the Web site to find a workshop in your area. www.cnvc.org/

Taber Shadburne—a phsychotherapist with advanced Buddhist training teaches kick-ass workshops on radical intimacy and relationship communication. He's based in the Bay area, but he teaches in various locations nationwide and over the phone. www.churchofsoul.org or www.lovewithoutlimits.com.

Cuddle Party—an organization that hosts nonsexual events geared at developing basic communication skills. www.cuddleparty.com

Appendix B

RELATIONSHIP AND SEXUALITY RESOURCES

SEXUALITY BOOKS, VIDEOS, AND WORKSHOPS

Brent, Bill. *The Ultimate Guide to Anal Sex for Men,* San Francisco: Cleis Press, 2002.

Hart, Jack. *Gay Sex: A Manual for Men Who Love Men.* New York: Alyson Books, 1998.

Michaels, Marcy and Marie DeSalle. *The Lowdown on Going Down: How to Give Her Mind-Blowing Oral Sex.* New York: Broadway Books, 2005.

Cage, Diana. *Box Lunch: The Layperson's Guide to Cunnilingus.* New York: Alyson Books, 2004.

Blue, Violet. *The Ultimate Guide to Cunnilingus: How To Go Down On a Woman and Give Her Exquisite Pleasure.* San Francisco: Cleis Press, 2002.

Silverstein, Charles. *The Joy of Gay Sex.* New York: HarperCollins, 2004.

Blue, Violet. *The Ultimate Guide to Fellatio: How To Go Down On a Man and Give Him Mind-Blowing Pleasure.* San Francisco: Cleis Press, 2002.

Lotney, Karolyn (a.k.a. Fairy Butch). *The Ultimate Guide to Strap-on Sex: A Complete Resource for Men and Women.* San Francisco: Cleis Press, 2000.

Chia, Mantak et al. *The Multi-Orgasmic Couple: Sexual Secrets Every Couple Should Know.* New York: HarperCollins, 2000.

Richardson, Diana. *The Heart of Tantric Sex: A Unique Guide to Love and Sexual Fulfillment.* Alresford, UK: O Books, 2003.

Anand, Margo. *The Art of Sexual Ecstasy: The Path of Sacred Sexuality for Western Lovers.* New York: Harper-Collins, 2003 (originally printed 1989).

Taormino, Tristan. *Down and Dirty Secrets: The New and Naughty Guide to Being Great in Bed.* New York: Regan Books, 2003.

Taormino, Tristan. *The Ultimate Guide to Anal Sex for Women.* San Francisco: Cleis Press, 1997.

The Kissing School—a Seattle-based kissing-education program hosts kissing workshops. Phone sessions available. 206-324-2526. www.kissingschool.com

Nina Hartley, porn actress and writer offers a series of sex how-to films. www.nina.com

The Human Awareness Institute—a San Francisco organization hosts workshops on intimacy, sexuality, and communication. www.hai.org. 415-571-5524

The San Francisco Sex Information Hotline—a free, anonymous, sex-positive information service, which offers nonjudgmental sex information and referrals. 415-989-7374

The Welcomed Consensus—a San Francisco–based organization that offers videos and courses on sensuality, relationships, communication, and lifestyles. The focus: better female orgasms. www.welcomed.com. 877-HOW-TO-DO

The Insight Institute—a group that offers workshops on sensuality, communication, and body-knowledge. www.insightinstitute.net

Esalen—an alternative education center that offers workshops on topics from massage to Tantra to "mindful loving." www.esalen.org

ALTERNATIVE RELATIONSHIP AND SEXUALITY BOOKS

Matik, Wendy-O. *Redefining Our Relationships: Guidelines for Responsible Open Relationships.* Oakland: Defiant Times Press, 2002.

Ravenscroft, Anthony. *Polyamory: Roadmaps for the Clueless & Hopeful.* Santa Fe: Crossquarter Publishing Group, 2004.

Anapol, Deborah, PhD. *Polyamory: The New Love Without Limits.* San Rafael, CA: IntiNet Resource Center, 1997.

Easton, Dossie and Catherine A. Liszt. *The Ethical Slut: A Guide to Infinite Sexual Possibilities.* San Francisco: Greenery Press, 1997.

Heinlein, Kris and Rozz Heinlein. *The Sex and Love Handbook: A Practical Optimistic Relationship Guide.* Do Things Records & Publishing, 2004.

Queen, Carol, PhD. *Real Live Nude Girl: Chronicles of Sex Positive Culture.* San Francisco: Cleis Press, 2002.

Daum, Megan. *My Misspent Youth: Essays.* New York: Open City Books, 2001. (Includes an essay on polyamory.)

Foster, Barbara, Michael Foster, and Letha Hadady. *Three In Love: Ménages à Trois from Ancient to Modern Times.* Backinprint.com, 1997.

Sincero, Jen. *The Straight Girl's Guide to Sleeping With Chicks.* New York: Fireside Books, 2005.

Labriola, Kathy. "Unmasking the Green-Eyed Monster: Managing Jealousy in Open Relationships," "Models of Open Relationships," and "Have You Considered Non-monogamy?" (Order free article copies by calling 510-841-5307.)

Kennedy, Elizabeth Lapovsky, and Madeline D. Davis. *Boots of Leather, Slippers of Gold: The History of a Lesbian Community.* New York: Penguin Books, 1994.

Smith-Rosenberg, Carroll. *Disorderly Conduct: Visions of Gender in Victorian America.* New York: Oxford University Press, 1985.

Chauncey, George. *Gay New York: Gender, Urban Culture, and the Making of the Gay Male World,* 1890–1940. New York: BasicBooks, 1994.

Garber, Marjorie. *Vice Versa: Bisexuality and the Eroticism of Everyday Life.* New York: Simon and Schuster, 1995.

D'Emilio, John, and Estelle B. Freedman. *Intimate Matters: A History of Sexuality in America.* New York: Perennial Library, 1989.

Rupp, Leila J. *A Desired Past: A Short History of Same-Sex Love in America.* Chicago: University of Chicago Press, 2002.

SEDUCTION RESOURCES

Strauss, Neil. *The Game: Penetrating the Secret Society of Pickup Artists.* New York: HarperCollins, 2005.

Mystery Method—a world-renowned pickup artist offers workshops and seminars on "natural game." www.mystery method.com

Stephan Hemon—a seduction guru who offers e-books, workshops, and lectures on "heart-centered pickup" (including three-way pickup), chakra balancing for seduction, and squirting orgasms. www.ideagasms.com

Charisma Sciences—a seduction-education company that holds seminars on natural charisma and body language. www.charismasciences.com

POLYAMORY AND THREESOMES IN FICTION

Heinlein, Robert. *Stranger in a Strange Land.* New York: Ace, 1961 (Reprinted, 1991). A 1961 utopian sci-fi novel, which popularized the concept of group marriage.

Bradley, Marion Zimmer. *The Forbidden Tower.* New York: DAW Books, 1977. A sci-fi novel featuring twin sisters in a group marriage.

Rimmer, Robert. *The Harrad Experiment.* Amherst, NY: Prometheus Books, 1973 (Reprinted, 1990). A novel on a sociological experiment in which students at a college live and sleep together in multiple arrangements.

Starhawk. *The Fifth Sacred Thing*. New York: Bantam Books, 1993. A novel about a conflict between a pagan polyamorous society in northern California and a fascist, fundamentalist Christian group from Southern California.

Kundera, Milan. *The Book of Laughter and Forgetting*. New York: Harper Perennial Modern Classics, 1991. (Originally published in Czech in 1979.) Mixing fiction, philosophy, and autobiography, one section involves a couple hiding their threesome from a visiting mother.

Hemingway, Ernest. *The Garden of Eden*. New York: Simon and Schuster, 1995 (originally published, 1986). A couple living on the French Riviera meet a young woman and fall in love with her.

Thirlwell, Adam. *Politics*. New York: HarperCollins, 2004. A novel about a threesome between two women and a man.

SEX SHOPS

Babeland

7007 Melrose Avenue
Los Angeles, CA 90038
323-634-9480

707 E Pike Street
Seattle, WA. 98122
206-328-2914

94 Rivington Street
New York, NY 10002
212-375-1701

43 Mercer Street
New York, N.Y. 10013
212-966-2120
www.babeland.com

Crimson Phoenix
2160 SE Ninety-sixth Avenue
Portland, OR 97216
503-228-0129
www.crimsonphoenix.org

Cupid's Treasure
3519 North Halsted Street
Chicago, IL 60657
773-348-3884

Dream Dresser Inc.
8444 Santa Monica Boulevard
West Hollywood, CA
323-848-3480

1042 Wisconsin Avenue, NW
Washington, DC 20007
202-625-0373

Eros Boutique
581A Tremont Street
Boston, MA 02118
617-425-0345
www.erosboutique.com

Eurotique
3109 Forty-fifth Street
West Palm Beach, FL 33407
800-486-9650
561-684-2302
www.eurotique.com

Eve's Garden
119 West 57th Street
Suite #420
New York, NY 10019
Telephone: 800-848-3837
Fax: 212-977-4306
www.evesgarden.com

Fantasy Unlimited
2027 Westlake Ave
Seattle, WA 98121
206-682-0167

Forbidden Fruit Toy Store
and Education Center
512 Neches Street
Austin, TX 78701
512-478-8358

Good Vibrations
603 Valencia Street
San Francisco, CA 94110
415-522-5460

1620 Polk Street
San Francisco, CA 94109
415-345-0400

2504 San Pablo Avenue
Berkeley, CA 94702
510-841-8987

308-A Harvard Street
Brookline, MA 02446
617-264-4400
www.goodvibes.com
1-800-BUY-VIBE

Intimacies
28 Center Street
Northampton, MA 01060
413-582-0709

It's My Pleasure
3106 NE 64th Avenue
Portland, OR 97213
503-280-8080

Passional
704 S Fifth Street
Philadelphia, PA 19147
215-829-4986
www.passional.net

Pleasure Chest
156 Seventh Avenue South
New York, NY 10014
212-242-2158

7733 Santa Monica Blvd.
West Hollywood, CA 90046
323-650-1022
www.thepleasurechest.com

Pleasure Place
1063 Wisconsin Avenue
Washington, DC 20007
202-333-8570

1710 Connecticut Avenue
Washington, DC 20009
202-483-3297
www.pleasureplace.com

Purple Passion
211 West 20th Street
New York, NY 10011
212-807-0486
www.purplepassion.com

Rubber Tree
4426 Burke Avenue North
Seattle, WA 98103
206-633-4750
www.rubbertree.org

Sh! Women's Erotic Emporium
57 Hoxton Square
London N1. 020-7613-5456
www.sh-womenstore.com

Spartacus Leathers
300 SW 12th Avenue
Portland, OR 97205
503-224-2604
www.spartacusleathers.com

Stormy Leather
1158 Howard Street
San Francisco, CA 94103
800-486-9650
415-626-1672
www.stormyleather.com

A Woman's Touch
600 Williamson Street
Madison, WI 53703
608-250-1928
www.a-womans-touch.com

BDSM ORGANIZATIONS AND CLUBS

The Spanking Club of New York

A social club that hosts events for heterosexual spankers in the New York area. www.scony.com

Eulenspiegel Society, New York, NY

The oldest and largest BDSM education and support group in the United States, founded in 1971. www.tes.org

Black Rose, Washington, DC

Black Rose is an organization that provides a forum for the many different expressions of power in love and play including: dominance & submission, bondage and discipline, fetishism, and cross-dressing. www.br.org

Threshold, Los Angeles, CA

Threshold is a nonprofit educational and support organization for adults (twenty-one and older) who have an interest in sadomasochism and other activities in a safe and consensual exchange of power. www.threshold.org

Society of Janus, San Francisco, CA

The Society of Janus is a San Francisco–based support and education group for people interested in learning about BDSM. Janus provides an opportunity to meet others with similar erotic interests in a safe, relaxed atmosphere. www.soj.org

The Next Generation of Chicago, Chicago, IL

The Next Generation of Chicago is a Chicago-based pansexual support, education, and social group for people age eighteen to thirty-five who are interested in BDSM. www.tgnc.org

POLYAMORY RESOURCES

The very helpful Chesapeake Polyamory Network offers a listing of regional polyamory groups across America. www.chespoly.org/docs/poly-groups.html

A Usenet newsgroup of polyamorists offers support, advice, and polyamory basics. http://www.polyamory.org

Live the Dream. An education and support group for people interested in polyamory. www.geocities.com/live_the_dream2000/index.html

Institute for Twenty-first Century Relationships. The Foundation of the National Coalition for Sexual Freedom. Aimed at educating and promoting a climate in which "all forms of ethical, consensual, and fulfilling relationship styles are broadly understood and are equally respected and honored as legitimate choices." www.lovethatworks.org

World Polyamory Association. A Hawaii-based organization, a network of polyamorists, which lists social events and workshops. www.worldpolyamoryassociation.com

Poly Matchmaker. An online dating service for those seeking all kinds of polyamorous relationships including:

vees, triads, open relationships, quads, networks, group marriage, multiple loves, polygyny, and polyandry. www.polymatchmaker.com

Polyamory Society. A nonprofit organization which promotes and supports the interest of individuals of multipartner relationships and families. www.polyamorysociety.org

Loving More magazine. The leading national magazine about ethical nonmonogamy. The Web site includes helpful links and a regional directory. www.lovemore.com

PolyFamilies. A support group for poly families. http://polyfamilies.com

Church of All Worlds—A neopagan church inspired by the science fiction novel *Stranger in a Strange Land* by Robert Heinlen, which "recognizes and blesses a variety of committed sacred sexual relationships as marriages." www.caw.org

Liberated Christians. A group for Christian polyamorists. www.libchrist.com

POLYAMORY AND OPEN RELATIONSHIP COUNSELORS, THERAPISTS, AND COACHES

Wendy-O Matik, author of *Redefining Our Relationships,* hosts workshops across the country on radically reinventing relationships. Check out her Web site for info: www.wendyomatik.com

An online region-specific guide to poly-friendly psychologists, therapists, and relationship counselors is available at http://www.polychromatic.com/pfp/psych.html

For a helpful article on what polyamory and mental health professionals should know about polyamory, check out www.polyamory.org/~joe/polypaper.htm

Deborah Anapol, PhD in clinical psychology, is the author of *Polyamory: The New Love Without Limits* and *Compersion: Using Jealousy as a Path to Unconditional Love.* She has been working with groups and individuals exploring conscious relating and sacred sexuality for over twenty years. She is a popular writer, leading edge teacher, relationship coach and practicing Tantrika. Her work has been featured on *Donahue, Sally Jesse Raphael, Real Sex,* and radio talk shows nationwide. Phone counseling available. www.lovewithout limits.com. 415-507-1739

Anita Wagner, a polyamory skills educator and director of outreach at the Institute for Twenty-first Century Relationships, is committed to helping others find happiness through responsible nonmonogamy. Phone counseling available. www.lovethatworks.org 703-561-8136

Robert McGarey, author of the Poly Communication Survival Kit and founder of the Center for Human Potential in Austin, offers personal growth sessions in person or over the phone for individuals, couples, triads, quads, or more-somes. www.humanpotentialcenter.org. 512-441-8988

Kathy Labriola provides low-fee counseling for individuals, couples, and groups. She has been counseling people in nontraditional relationships for more than twenty-five years. She also facilitates discussion and support groups on open relationships. She is available for phone counseling sessions. For further information or to receive free educational pamphlets on ethical non-monogamy, call 510-841-5307

Kamala Devi is a gifted life coach who specializes in alternative relationship coaching and sacred sexuality. Phone sessions available. www.partnerplayshop.com and www.blisscoach.com

Geri Weitzman, PhD, is a licensed psychologist in the Bay area, who specializes in alternative relationships, codependency, personal growth, self-acceptance, coming out, bisexuality, and polyamory. Phone counseling available. www.numenor.org/~gdw/psychologist. 415-517-7965

ALTERNATIVE LIFESTYLE RESOURCES

Lifestyle Lounge. A fee-based Web site featuring personal ads, a chat room, regional event listings, and exclusive swinger-oriented vacations. www.lifestylelounge.com

Swing Clubs USA. Features lifestyle event listings. www.swingclubs.us/

North American Swing Club Association. www.nasca.com

Cake. A community that throws female-oriented sex parties featuring burlesque routines, lingerie, hipster porn, and more. www2.cakenyc.com

Kinky Salon—A San Francisco–based community dedicated to sex-positive self expression. www.kinkysalon. com

LUST Erotic Dance Parties. Selective and exclusive members-only parties with DJs, music, and entertainment in luxurious settings and locations in and around Los Angeles and Las Vegas. www.lustparty.com

Wilkinson Photography. LosAngeles–based alternative lifestyle photography and fine-art erotica, offers photography for singles, couples, and threesomes. Sexy pics are a must for online personal ads. Photo shoots in other cities available. www.photosbywilkinson.com

NOTES

1. The astrology section relies on Judith Bennet, *Sex Signs* (New York: St. Martin's Griffin, 1980); Martine, *Sexual Astrology: A Sign-By-Sign Guide to Your Sensual Stars,* (New York: Random House, 1976); and Judy Hall, *Sun Signs for Lovers:The Astrological Guide to Love, Sex and Relationships* (London: Octopus Publishing Group, 2005).

2. According to a report presented by psychologist Dr. Weitzman at the Annual Diversity Conference of the Division of Counseling Psychology at the University of Albany, in 1999. A study by Rubin & Adams (1986)

found no significant difference in marital stability between couples with open relationships compared to monogamous couples.

3. Gross, Jane. "Does She Speak for Today's Women?—Patricia Ireland, President of NOW," *New York Times,* March 1, 1992, sec. 6, Late Edition.

4. This section was informed by Kathy Labriola's article, "Unmasking the Green-Eyed Monster: Managing Jealousy in Open Relationships" and Dr. Deborah Anapol's *Polyamory: The New Love Without Limits.*

5. The section on healthy and unhealthy reasons for monogamy and nonmonogamy was informed by an interview with relationship counselor, Kathy Labriola.

6. Yoshino, Kenjo. "The Epistemic Contract of Bisexual Erasure," *Stanford Law Review,* v. 52, No. 2, 2000.

7. George Chauncey, *Gay New York: Gender, Urban Culture, and the Making of the Gay Male World, 1890–1940* (New York: Basicbooks, 1994).

8. Stephanie Coontz, *The Way We Never Were: American Families and the Nostalgia Trap* (New York, 2000), p. 66; Other historians who cover romantic friendships include:

Carroll Smith-Rosenberg, *Disorderly Conduct: Visions of Gender in Victorian America* (New York, 1985); John D'Emilio and Estelle B. Freedman, *Intimate Matters: A History of Sexuality in America* (New York, 1989); Lillian Faderman, *Surpassing the Love of Men: Romantic Friendship and Love Between Women from the Renaissance to the Present* (New York, 1981).

9. This section was informed by Kathy Labriola's article, "Models of Open Relationships."

10. This section on coming out was informed by interviews with relationship counselors Kathy Labriola.

ACKNOWLEDGMENTS

These are some of the amazing people I'm super grateful to for helping me out:

Lukas Volgar, Don Weise, and everyone else at Avalon for making this book possible. Paul Levine for having faith in this project from the beginning and Kaya Dzankich for illustrating with enthusiasm.

All the friends and family members who answered my probing questions about their sex lives without raising an eyebrow. My ever-supportive sister for asking thoughtful questions and offering insightful comments (instead of freaking out). She's infinitely awesome. MF, my dear wheel of fortune, for making me laugh my ass off every day and showing me how to seduce anyone, armed with nothing but a martini and taffeta fish costume. Her ridiculous charm and buoyant optimism bring oodles of happiness into my life.

My friends from Hedgebrook for hilarious (and candid) dinner conversations about sex and relationships. B-sides for teaching me that it's fun to be aggressively unsexy and to the mermaid-school crew for teaching me just how fun sexy can be. R, whose infectious curiosity kept me up all night and opened a new world to me. Also, BB, LG, KB, JenDes, SK, SM, SB, LK, DK, JM, FV, Kel, Abby, Ian, and KP—who gave me all kinds of love along the way.

Kamala for showing me that being a misfit can be a spiritual calling and for magically transforming my neuroses into purposeful action. Her genius way of inspiring others to live big is beyond dazzling, and I couldn't have met her at a better time.

Everyone out there who shared intimate details of their relationships and sex lives with me. This book couldn't have been written without their insights and honesty. Beyond taking the time to share what they've learned from their own experiences in unconventional relationships, many of these people also invited me into their lives and welcomed me to use their circles for my research experiments. Not only did they provide backbone information for this book, but also they showed me that there are lots and lots of people out there chucking mainstream sex and romance structures and finding their own revolutionary ways to make love work. Their guts and grace blow me away.

And, finally, M, my sweet coadventurer in love and life. Even though this book wasn't his cup of tea, he was supportive from the beginning and was always there when I needed him with encouragement, egg sandwiches, and a brutally-honest critical eye. His patience, humor, openness to change, and super-human ability to love me without crushing me, continues to amaze me. I feel enormously lucky to be sharing this journey with him.

I'm hugely grateful. Thank you!

ABOUT THE AUTHOR

Vicki Vantoch is an award-winning sex and gender historian, journalist, and threesome enthusiast. She has written on subjects ranging from underground art scenes to fingernail fashion to postwar airline stewardesses. Her work has appeared in publications such as the *Washington Post, U.S. News & World Report,* and the *Los Angeles Times.* Vantoch received a B.A. in anthropology from the University of Chicago and an M.A. from the University of Southern California, where she is he is currently completing her PhD in the history of gender and sexuality. A recipient of numerous prestigious awards and fellowships including a Guggenheim Fellowship and NASA's Aerospace History Fellowship, Vantoch has lectured on sex and gender topics at venues across the nation including the Smithsonian Institution and the Library of Congress.